COMPLETELY UNAUTHORIZED

THE MYTH OF
LOST

Solving the Mysteries and Understanding the Wisdom

MARC OROMANER

iUniverse, Inc.
New York   Bloomington

The Myth of *Lost*
Solving the Mysteries and Understanding the Wisdom

iUniverse books may be ordered through booksellers or by contacting:

iUniverse
1663 Liberty Drive
Bloomington, IN 47403
www.iuniverse.com
1-800-Authors (1-800-288-4677)

ISBN: 978-0-595-48456-0 (pbk)
ISBN: 978-0-595-48991-6 (cloth)
ISBN: 978-0-595-60550-7 (ebk)

Printed in the United States of America

CONTENTS

Acknowledgments

So many bizarre events occurred at just the right time to make this book a reality, and for that, I guess I need to thank the mysterious powers of the universe. First, it arranged it so that I would continually catch intriguing episodes of *Lost*, enticing me to watch. When that didn't work, it then used its henchmen to try to convince me of the show's brilliance. These destiny guides materialized in the form of friends and co-workers—most notably, Eileen Connell and Brad Eisenstein, who were both incredulous that someone of my spiritually-obsessed caliber did not watch the show and insisted that I immediately begin doing so. Their attempts failed, due mostly to a really big book I was working on that had severely limited my free time. Therefore, the universe decided to help out by giving me lots of free time. It did this by causing the computer I was using to write my book, to die. While I was in the process of getting a new one, Brad lent me his *Lost—The Complete First Season* DVDs. After about three episodes, I was hooked.

My friend Scott Schwartz deserves thanks, not only for watching most of the *Lost* episodes with me, but for putting up with my obsessive rewinding and freeze-framing of various scenes—even before I had decided to write the book.

For providing valuable feedback on an early incarnation of *The Myth of Lost*, I am very grateful to my brother, David, and my friend and former co-worker Jennifer Daniels. Thanks also to fellow TV book author, Tripp Whetsell, for his marketing advice and suggestion to shorten the book's title, which was originally: *The Myth of Lost: Solving the mysteries of the hit ABC TV show and understanding how its wisdom can provide valuable insight into the meaning of our lives.* Just kidding; it was never quite that long, but it was close.

Then there's a whole list of people I need to thank for their talents and expertise that helped make this book a reality. This includes (but is not limited to) my publishing attorney, Alan J. Kaufman, Esq.; everyone who pitched in at iUniverse, particularly, Brenda Kluck, Kelli Shute, and Jason Straw; the many editors, most notably, Melissa Watkins Starr, who worked diligently to translate my manuscript into something resembling English; and Jimmy Ng, my friend and co-worker who not only created a surrealistically cool cover design but accommodated my desire to have lots of hidden images for readers to uncover. Production master Andrew Addino also deserves recognition for his help with the book's plethora of marketing materials (you are going to help me, right Andrew?)

I absolutely have to thank all the *Lost* fans out there who inspired me to write this book, especially those who contributed to Web sites, blogs, and podcasts that triggered my imagination and my memory, helping me to recall the thousands of minute details about the show.

This book's acknowledgments page would not be complete without thanking the shamanic creators and producers of *Lost,* particularly J.J. Abrams, Damon Lindelof, and Carlton Cuse. They have inspired millions of couch potatoes to become active participants in solving the mystery of a TV show, and in so doing, have reenergized our desire to solve the mysteries of the world around us. While they might not realize it, I believe their contributions will help guide this world in a more enlightened direction—depending, of course, on what their ending for the show turns out to be. Regardless of the ending, however, I'd like to think that *Lost* has inspired new hope for a whole new beginning for all of us.

Finally, for all their support, I am tremendously grateful to my friends, family, and everyone who followed along with my progress while I was working on the book—even though most of them didn't even watch the show it was based on. Your energy not only helped me overcome many challenges, it also helped convince the universe to bring about the writer's strike, which bought me the extra time I needed to get this book out there. As *Lost* teaches us, everything happens for a reason.

Preface

Like all great mythology, *Lost* reveals hidden truths about the inner workings of our world. Somewhere, deep within our subconscious, we know what these truths are. When we hear them—even when they're disguised as mythology—they resonate with us, creating an incredible vibration that makes us feel enlightened. In other words, *Lost* is more than just a show. It's a microcosm of the real world. How the series ends isn't nearly as important as what it is teaching us in its weekly episodes. *Lost* is perhaps one of the greatest psychological experiments ever conducted on a mass of people simultaneously, and this fact just might end up playing into the resolution of its storyline. While I don't believe that this "audience is the experiment" direction is where the show is heading; if it is, it definitely could result in an eye-opening and unexpected conclusion. For this ending, it would turn out that the TV audience has been part of the *Lost* experiment all along—an experiment designed to teach the world that we are all connected, that we should look for clues in the universe, and that everything happens for a reason.

At the very least, *Lost* has been hugely influential in getting jaded TV viewers interactively involved in a show, as its many clues encourage them to search the Internet for answers. For these reasons and many more, *Lost* has ushered in a new era of TV programming—one where we are active participants in what we are watching. Acknowledging these many influences, the last episode in the scenario previously described would have the cast coming out of character to thank the audience for taking part in the greatest worldwide experiment ever conducted. Of course, some fans will be absolutely crushed if this turns out to be the ending. Personally, I would love it. Because watching the show, I wanted to be a part of it. I wanted to be stuck on that island with Kate, Shannon, Claire, and ... well, mostly just them. This ending would make me part of that world. As satisfying as this solution would be, however, I sincerely doubt that it actually will be used to conclude the show. Since coming up with it, though, I have developed another solution that makes much more sense and remains within the context of *Lost*'s mythology. This more developed solution is the one that's used throughout most of this book.

According to the wisdom of *Lost* and many other myths, everything happens for a reason. That being the case, since you've stumbled upon this book, there's most likely some information in it you're meant to find. While I had nothing to do with creating the show, I did feel a very real connection with it, like it was speaking to me ... personally. I guess you felt the same way. I'd just like you to know what I know—or at least *think* I know—about *Lost* and what it's all about. I strongly believe that whatever creative force its creators plugged into, I've tapped into as well. I know this because of a novel I'd just completed writing several months before I began watching the show. Some of the plot elements and twists in *Lost* were so similar to what happened in my book, it was uncanny.

There are two main reasons I decided to write *The Myth of Lost*. First, I'd been disappointed by the endings of various sci-fi movies and TV series before, usually because I felt the writers lost touch with the soul of the story. I'm not sure if it's because of the plethora of film classes I took in college, my dabbling in the mystical teachings of Kabbalah, or just the way my brain is wired, but I tend to be pretty good at recognizing the way a story needs to go in order to be spiritually fulfilling. While *Lost*'s first two seasons seemed completely on track, with the start of its third season, I began getting concerned. I felt that the story was drifting away from the myth and becoming increasingly convoluted. Interestingly, it was right at this time that I had an epiphany about a solution to all the mysteries of the show. Even if it wasn't the same one envisioned by *Lost*'s creators, it provided a very fulfilling and surprisingly simple resolution to the series. As a devoted fan, I quickly realized that if someone else had come up with this same theory, I'd desperately want to know what it was. So, I decided to share this one with anyone who'd be interested in it.

As I began to flesh out the details, however, another—perhaps more meaningful—reason emerged. I realized that the book wanted to be about more than just a solution to a mysterious TV show. It wanted to be about the solution to your life, which may be even more important depending on what you plan on doing with this information. If you think about it, your life is like *Lost* in a lot of ways: it has a beginning, a middle, and an end; it has a bunch of characters who have some major issues; it has a lot of weird stuff that doesn't seem to make any sense; it has challenges—its ups, its downs, its surprises you didn't see coming; and it has a whole bunch of hotties you ain't ever gonna have sex with. More relevant, however, the show is governed by principles that seem vaguely familiar—almost as though they are the very same principles our lives are governed by. Yet most of us aren't petting imaginary horses, seeing the same set of random numbers everywhere, or being picked up and smashed into a tree by a gigantic smoke monster—so what does it all mean? That's what this book is about.

Using *Lost*'s characters, themes, and mysteries as a template, this book will illustrate how a seemingly baffling show can make sense out of life. Best of all, you don't even have to be a die-hard fan of the show to get it. Completed after the end of *Lost*'s third season, the book provides the gist of the basics so casual viewers, newbies, and even *Lost* dropouts will all be able to follow along. Regardless of your devotion to *Lost*, though, you'll probably want to check out missed episodes and begin watching the show more regularly after reading this book. That's just my little thank-you to the creators for coming up with such an enlightening TV experience—one which by now you must be dying to know the meaning of. So without further ado, let's get to it. Are you excited? I can't hear you—I said *are you excited??* Okay, I still can't hear you, but let's just move on.

Why *Lost* Is Alive

onsidering that I'm a pretty big fan of science fiction, having grown up with old *Twilight Zone* and *Star Trek* reruns as well as being a pretty regular *X-Files* fanatic, I guess it's pretty odd that I didn't have much of an interest in *Lost* when ABC first aired it on September 22, 2004. Perhaps, having recently come off the disappointing last two years of *X-Files*, I just didn't feel like getting involved in another one-hour sci-fi drama that would only let me down in the end. A one-hour show is a pretty big commitment, and since this one starred that guy from *Party of Five*, I figured it would end up being nothing more than a typical, made-for-TV movie. Boy, was I wrong.

In spite of my misgivings, I somehow managed to catch five minutes of the *Lost* premiere. I think it was when the monster was roaming about. Now, I like monsters. But the fact that this one was invisible didn't speak too highly of the show's budget. (I'd missed the million-dollar airplane wreckage scene that had eaten up most of it, leaving nothing for anything else). So I began channel surfing and probably ended up on some *Seinfeld* rerun—probably the one about going with the opposite of all your instincts.

Fast forward to May 25, 2005. By this point, I had totally forgotten about the show. I'd hear people talking about it from time to time, but I'd also hear about Paris Hilton's *The Simple Life*, too, so I wasn't particularly concerned. Then, after managing to miss all but five minutes of *Lost*'s first season, I once again stumbled upon an important episode—the season finale. Just as I tuned in, some adolescent kid was getting abducted from a boat by what appeared to be the Gorton's fisherman. Not surprisingly, this was not enough to convince me of the show's brilliance.

While I'm pretty sure ABC ran *Lost* reruns over the summer, I didn't catch another episode until the second series premiere. I caught it right from the beginning. But having not seen much of the series, I had absolutely no idea what was going on when some hippie-haired dude woke up, put on some cheesy '70s record, injected himself with some vitamins or something, and began to punch seemingly random numbers into a computer. Little did I realize that no one else had any idea what was going on at that point either.

The universe was really slapping me around by this point—trying to get me to start watching the show—but alas, I continued to turn the other cheek. That is, until the next time I caught an episode. It was the second season finale, and I caught a good three-quarters of it. Weird, how I kept seeing only the important episodes. This time, I got sucked in, watched it to the end, and regretted having not gotten involved in the show earlier. But not so much that I actually wanted to go back and watch them all.

Coincidentally, though, my creative director at work had just completed watching the first season *Lost* DVDs he'd purchased and asked if I'd be interested in borrowing them. Twenty-four episodes? I had no time for such frivolous pursuits! I was in the middle of self-editing a thousand-page book I'd just written that I hoped would one day save the world! Fortunately, the universe had other plans for me and decided that this would be a perfectly good time for my nine-year-old Mac to die. While I waited to get a new one, along with all new software, I had some time to kill. So I figured I'd follow the clues of my own life. *Lost* finally had me right where it wanted me—pinned to the ground under its huge, hairy buttocks.

After I'd finished watching the first season, a co-worker happened to mention that he'd recorded all of the second season episodes to DVD and wondered if I might want to borrow them. Okay, now the universe was just being blatantly obvious. I succumbed and once again decided to take delight in the sweet, sweet nectar that is surely a severe

Lost addiction. Unlike Charlie, I just couldn't throw those heroin-filled Virgin Mary statues away.

I finished the second season a couple weeks before season three was scheduled to begin. Not only would this be my first time watching a full episode along with the rest of the viewers in the Eastern Standard Time zone, enabling me to share in the collective *Lost* experience, it would also be the first time I would have to actually deal with commercials. Being that I worked in advertising and was surrounded by ads all day long, this was not something I was looking forward to. Even so, I was able to pull myself together and mentally prepare myself for the challenge. If I'd learned anything from *Lost*, it was to always face your worst adversary head-on with no fear.

After many restless nights—I was having dreams about being stuck on the island, and Sawyer kept calling me Fro-jo on account of my curly hair—at last the day of *Lost's* return arrived! It was Wednesday, October 4, 2006, and celestialweather.com had this to say about the planetary alignment that night:

Now in Pisces, the moon continues to shine dream-light on the world. She passes exactly over Uranus at 8:20 PM in a moment that may bring sudden empathy or recognition of a hidden connection.

Recognition of a hidden connection? Woo-hoo! What I didn't realize at the time was how prophetic that prediction truly was. After watching the show, which I thought was pretty decent, but certainly not one of the better episodes, I felt something swimming around my brain that I didn't know quite what to make of. As a writer who's— how should I put this?—a tad insane, I experience this sensation rather frequently, so didn't give it much thought.

Later that night, however, I had a revelation. An epiphany. I was eating a midnight snack of Frosted Flakes when it suddenly dawned on me! Yes! Everything made complete sense—the monster, the numbers, the hatches, the Others, even the tropical polar bears—it all fit together! I'd solved it! And it was great! I loved it! But what if it wasn't the solution that the writers had in mind? I'd come up with interesting ideas involving the *Star Wars* prequels and *Matrix* sequels, and in those cases, I was severely let down by what ended up on the screen. No! I would not let it happen again! This time I would share the fulfilling ending with the world—the ending that the universe intended us to hear—whether the creators knew it or not.

When Shamans Lose Their Way

The solution contained in this book most likely won't end up being exactly like what the show's creators have in mind for *Lost*. In fact, it might not even end up resembling their solution in the least. Doesn't matter. Why? To understand that, you first need to understand why certain stories strike a chord with society, while others completely fall flat. In a nutshell, successful stories all do one thing: they reveal hidden truths about the way the world really works. While we all have access to these truths, they're hidden deep within humanity's collective unconsciousness. Once we begin to hear them, however, they resonate with a part of us that had been forgotten, creating a beautiful vibration that just feels right.

Star Wars did this for a lot of people—a story about how a simple farm boy with big dreams goes through a series of challenges to unlock his destiny, using a mysterious force in the universe to help guide him to success. In case you didn't know, the simple farm boy is *you* (whether you're simple, have ever worked on a farm, or for that matter, are even a boy). We all have longings to play our part in the universe, so that movie resonated with society and created a sensation.

Lost is yet another example of a story that is trying to tell us something without shoving it in our face and making it obvious. Usually, a good myth will disguise the truth it's based upon. It does this because the rational, conscious mind isn't what's aware of this truth—

5

the *unconscious* mind is. So, in order to reach that part of you, the story must speak a language that can sneak past your logical, thinking brain and head down to the cellar of your deeper consciousness. Not only do all good stories do this, all good art does this as well.

The language of the universe is much too complicated for our itty-bitty human brains to comprehend. That's why it must speak to us through channels that go *beyond* what we can fully comprehend. The universe imparts wisdom that isn't apparent on the surface, but can only be found between the lines. This is the realm of symbolism and metaphor. It is the realm of the artist, storyteller, and poet. Yet often these creatives themselves don't even fully understand the very messages they are relaying to us mere mortals, for they are only doing their jobs as channelers. Without this understanding, the conscious, rational mind—and ego—of these channelers will usually interfere with the purity of the message they are meant to convey. This leaves the message muddy at best, and completely warped at worst, explaining much of the confusion we are experiencing in our society today. If only our mythological delivery system could be as pure as it used to be.

Not too long ago, most of mankind lived in tribes or clans. In order to survive, it was extremely important for people to be able to get along with the environment in which they lived. The problem was that mankind didn't always know the best way to go about doing this. Luckily (though, according to the wisdom of *Lost*, it probably wasn't just luck), certain tribesmen were born with or developed magical abilities that enabled them to interpret the supernatural energies of the universe for the rest of their fellow tribesmen to understand. Perhaps even more fortunate, in cases where these abilities were not inherited or brought about through some sort of illness or trauma, they could often be learned with intense training. However they came upon their abilities, the magical tribesmen who had them were known as shamans, and they would often gather their clan around a fire and explain mysteries in the guise of stories. Members of the clan would then pass down these stories from generation to generation, creating legends of their people. Many of these stories form the mythology that has become the foundation of just about every classically themed story we tell today. Truth be told, these ancient myths are all ingrained in our collective psyches.

Really, there are no new myths. Only new ways of telling them, using modern scenarios that are easier for us to relate to. *Star Wars* is the same myth as *King Arthur,* which is the same myth as *Aladdin,* which is the same myth as *The Odyssey,* which is the same myth as David and Goliath. In all these tales, one individual must call upon their inner strength to fight the odds and, with the aid of a special weapon, conquer a powerful evil so that they can bring peace to the land. Similarly, *Lost* is based on the same myth as *The Matrix,* which is the same myth as *The Wizard of Oz,* which is the same myth as *Alice in Wonderland,* which is the same myth as the ancient Greek philosopher, Plato's "Allegory of the Cave" from his work, *The Republic.* These myths illustrate that life is an illusion that requires us to go on a quest to discover who we really are and that we can go home at any time simply by waking up to this truth. (Just click your heels together, Dorothy.) Interestingly, this is also the same myth as that of the Messiah, a.k.a. Neo, a.k.a. the Wizard, and a.k.a. the White Rabbit ("I'm late! I'm late!"). In *Lost,* the messianic archetype is known as "Him." And "Him" is he who will awaken the lost gang to their truth if the show's creators know what they are doing. This brings me back to why they may not.

When George Lucas wrote *Star Wars,* he was channeling the myth of the coming spiritual awaking which resonated with an entire generation that is now helping to bring it about. When he wrote the three prequels, however, he was telling more of a political allegory (i.e., *Gulliver's Travels,* which is about the incessant bickering of humanity and all its stupid rules and laws) than a great mythical truth. Episodes I-III of the *Star Wars* saga tell the tale of what happens when culture gets so caught up in propaganda, bureaucracy, and what it views as morality, that it turns a blind eye as a madman rises to power with hopes of taking over the world. Now, I have no doubt whatsoever as to why George Lucas was channeling this story when he was—it was a moral lesson that society needed to hear to warn us about the times in which we currently live. I just don't think it was a message on par with the original *Star Wars,* especially since it ended on a negative note for the hero. A true myth should never do that. The aim of the myth is to uplift and inspire. Taken as a whole, all six *Star Wars* episodes do this, but the first three episodes just don't do it as well. They focus more on special effects than story, and this was why there was such a backlash after they came out. There are a number of simple changes these films could have undergone that would have made them as powerful as the earlier films, but that's a discussion for another book. My point is that sometimes shamans lose their way.

That's right: artists, writers, and poets are, in effect, modern day shamans. The only difference is, instead of sitting around a flickering fire to experience their stories, we now view them from the flickering light of movie screens or TV sets. We still prefer to be in the dark to receive our myths—partly because we've been doing it for thousands of years and it has become ingrained in our psyches, and partly because being in the dark matches our state of mind before we are enlightened.

The Matrix trilogy is the perfect example of a story in which the shaman lost his way. The reason the first movie was such a success was because it accurately updated the Messiah/Life-As-Illusion myth in a creative and interesting way that hadn't been done before. We were left wondering, "What if life really was just a computer program?" Pretty cool thought. The second and third *Matrix* movies, however, got too caught up in fighting and special effects to continue the myth. The way the trilogy ended—and sorry for ruining it, but trust me, I'm not spoiling anything that was worth seeing—Neo made a deal with the computers so they wouldn't pick on the helpless rebel humans anymore. They promised to leave the rebels in peace in their little underground misery known as Zion while the rest of humanity continued its oblivious existence in the matrix. This sends out the message that mankind will never be free from the illusion. Nobody wants to hear that. Like Lucas, the creators of *Matrix* got too caught up in an allegory for the current state of affairs and not the hope—the myth—we are all meant to strive for.

If the writers of *The Matrix* had continued with the myth, it would have ended with Neo sacrificing himself to the evil computer virus known as Agent Smith. Once this happened, all of Neo's energy would have been sucked into Smith and spread to all of his victims—which was basically all of humanity by that point. And since Neo was aware of the Truth, his energy should have served to wake up everybody from the Matrix illusion. Every human on Earth, given the energy of Neo, should have broken free from the Matrix's hold on them and woken from their pods as Neo had in the first film. Imagine, an angelic choir singing as the entire human race finally starts to wake up—confused—

and pull out their plugs! Without the power from these human minds, the machines in the real world would have run out of juice, causing them to freeze in their tracks, saving Zion and all the rebel humans outside the illusionary matrix. The film would have then concluded with the underground Zion inhabitants coming to the surface, the smoke clearing, and billions of enlightened humans emerging from their life-long confinement in the illusionary world. At last, a new world could now begin, fulfilling the Messiah/rebirth cycle myth.

I'm sure that everyone would have liked the ending of the *Matrix* trilogy a whole lot better had it concluded this way. It's a much more inspiring message than the actual ending, which had mankind continuing to live in the illusion under the shadow of the machines, as we do now. Just as in the movie, the money and spectacle of our illusionary, material world defeated the message we were meant to hear. In other words, the bad guys won. That's why we all walked out of the final *Matrix* with a bad feeling in the pit of our stomach—something was off. The movie had lost its soul—the powerful myth of the first movie. That's why it totally fell flat.

As for *Lost*, I'm getting a bit concerned. Having already been disappointed with *Star Wars* and *The Matrix,* I'd hate to have my dreams smashed to pieces yet again with what is a truly great mythic TV show—especially since it involves such a greater time commitment. That's why I'm attempting to nip it in the bud, getting the message out there just in case the writers have lost their way. So far, I don't think they have. So there's still time. However, there is reason to worry. The universe (the island) has tipped me off. Beginning with the early episodes of the third season, the artistic integrity of the writers began to get compromised by network pressure for ratings. This was why *Lost* started looking more like a soap opera than a great mythic show. Look, if we want to see senseless violence and gratuitous sex based around a thinly veiled excuse for a plot, there are countless other television programs to choose from. Bring back the myth of the show, I say! This is only one of the reasons I began to get worried. There were other hints as well from as early as the first season.

Like most people who watch *Lost,* I was always on the lookout for clues. And when I reached the episode where Charlie's band, Driveshaft, sings their infamous one-hit-wonder, I'd thought for sure

I'd found another one. Only problem was, I'd misheard the lyrics. Ironically though, my version actually made more sense and was more in line with the myth. I *thought* the title of Driveshaft's song was "You Are Everybody." Another clue to be sure. This title not only fits in with the recurring *Lost* theme of all the characters being connected to one another, as illustrated in flashbacks which reveal how the lives of the castaways were often intertwined before they'd ever met, it also fits with the mythic message of the show—that *all of us* are connected.

It wasn't until I reached the end of the first season DVD set, however, that I discovered the horrific truth. Included on the compilation was a bonus disc which revealed how the title for the Driveshaft song came about. Turned out that one of the *Lost* creators had picked it up from the rantings of an angry audience member on an old episode of *Donahue,* and it had become something of an inside joke amongst the *Lost* crew. "You all everybody acting like it's stupid people wearing expensive clothes!" is what the woman apparently said. And that line became the chorus for the Driveshaft song—"You *All* Everybody," as in "y'all everybody," not "You *Are* Everybody" as I had mistakenly assumed.

Why had the show creator, Damon Lindelof, witnessed this outburst, and why had it struck him so funny that it had stayed in his mind all these years? Was it so that Driveshaft could have that exact line as the title for their song? Or was he meant to translate it using his shamanic superpowers into something more appropriate for the myth of the show? Methinks the latter was more likely the case. Lindelof missed a golden opportunity to add to the mystique of *Lost* by, instead, poking fun at an obviously uneducated woman's shortcomings. Is it any accident that the name "Damon" is a variant of "Damian"—the child of Satan who starred in the *Omen* films? I'll leave that up to you to decide.

Okay, that was all a bit tongue-in-cheek, but little clues like these are often indicators of larger truths. Just as how a single droplet of water contains the same reflection as a huge lake, so too does a small truth reflect a big one. Little things mean a lot. Similarly, it has been said that "how you do anything is how you do everything." So if the show creators are missing some of the smaller truths when writing the smaller plot points, chances are they are probably also missing some of the bigger truths when writing the bigger plot points. In other words, they might not be fully tapping into the collective truth that *Lost* is based on, and therefore they may be misinterpreting some of it.

Case in point: the way the *Lost* pilot was originally written, Jack was meant to be killed by the monster at the end of the two-hour episode. The writers did this because they wanted to break the old *Star Trek* Red Shirt Rule which stated that the show's main characters could never be harmed. Only new characters, who always wore red shirts on *Star Trek* to signify their lowly ensign ranks, were expendable. Boone actually mentions the phenomenon in one of the later *Lost* episodes. Problem is, most everyone who read about the Jack-dying scenario *hated* it. Why? Because we identify with the heroes of stories. We are meant to live vicariously through their adventures. A hero can't die before his or her adventure has even begun. We are left without anyone to identify with, breaking our connection to what's going on. The hero is meant to inspire. He *can* be killed, but only if he dies fighting for what he believed in, as William Wallace does in *Braveheart*. Otherwise, what's the message? That we should give up before we even try? Who wants to hear that? It goes against the myth. Yes, the whole Red Shirt Rule is cheesy, but you know what? It works. These days, it's better to make it less predictable than the obvious *Star Trek* way, but the rule should still be more or less in place. The writers, in trying to shake things up a bit and leave audiences utterly lost, were being too subversive—leaving the truth of the story almost unrecognizable. After realizing their mistake, the scene was rewritten to have the plane's pilot get killed by the monster instead, leaving the classic aspects of the myth in tact. Had this not been done, *Lost* would have very likely been cancelled after the first few episodes. Interestingly, Greg Grunberg, the actor playing the pilot, who sacrificed his role for the good of the show, went on to play one of the heroes in the popular NBC show, *Heroes*. Just as his character followed the path dictated by the rules of mythology, so too did his real life.

While I respect the show creators for trying to go against the predictable formula, there's a reason that formula is in place and has been for thousands of years—it works. When we experience a story, *we* are the heroes. We are the ones who are meant to rise up and face our fears in our own lives, and, of course, we are meant to succeed. This is what good stories inspire us to do. That's why they make us feel good—they're getting in touch with our soul. But the show creators almost blew it. Yet again, another hint that they might not be totally on track with the mythic message they are translating for us in *Lost*. Admittedly, it's easy to get distracted from the message when you have deadlines, executive pressures, and many writers working on one story. Not to mention a story that has to go on and on and on and still keep audiences involved week after week. There's also temptation in the form of sex, violence, and special effects. Hopefully, network TV and budgetary restraints will prevent *Lost* from wasting too much energy in these areas. But it can still end up missing the myth if the writers get too caught up in details to lose us on the big message. Shaking things up a bit is fine, and *Lost* writers have kept it interesting by killing off major characters like Boone, Ana Lucia, Mr. Eko, and Charlie. They just shouldn't go overboard, or else they risk sacrificing the show's mythic message in favor of an attempt at originality that doesn't ring true for anyone watching.

Myths in the Media

I've been throwing around the term "myth" a lot without having really explained what a myth is. In layman's terms, a myth is a story that attempts to explain the mysteries of the universe using characters and situations we can understand. For example, there are no myths involving radioactive quarks residing in the pseudo-stratified, glandular, columnar, ciliated, epithelial tissue of a dead Australopithecus-afarensis's doppelgänger floating near Rigel Kentaurus, because no one could understand that. Usually, when we think of myths, we think of the stories of the ancient Greeks or of some "primitive" tribe somewhere in Africa. Truth is, we're still creating myths to explain our world to this very day and incorporating the message of older ones into our modern ideas about life.

Technically, our Bible—the good book that we base much of our culture on—fits the definition of a myth. That isn't to say that it isn't true—some myths such as Robin Hood or King Arthur may be based on true events—just that it's a story that serves to explain why we're here that features the exploits of heroes, villains, and supernatural beings. To be fair, the Koran, the Torah, and the Book of Mormon are also myths. Ironically, *Dianetics* is not a myth in the traditional sense because it is a set of ideas and practices, not a story with gods and monsters. Then again, using another definition of myth, "any invented story, idea, or concept,"[1] *Dianetics* would then be classified as a myth by everyone except for devout Scientologists.

Along with our religious texts, our fables, tall tales, fairytales, comic book stories, and sci-fi movies are all also myths. For example, Superman is most often thought of as a Messianic myth. Krypton resident Jor-El, whose name in Hebrew can translate to "light of God," sends his only son, Kal-El[2], or "voice of God"[3] to Earth so that he may be its savior. Sound familiar? Little Kal-el, whose name in his native Kryptonian apparently translates to "star-child,"[4] is found by Martha and Jonathan (Mary and Joseph) Kent, who decide that their huge farmhouse is too small for the baby boy so he's kept in a barn (stable).

So if Superman is a myth, what is its most recent adaptation, *Superman Returns,* telling us? Well, I'm going to have to give away a spoiler to reveal that. In the movie, we discover that Superman (the modern mythological representation of Jesus) had a child. What's particularly interesting about this revelation is that it comes at a time when, thanks to *The Da Vinci Code*, mankind is beginning to believe that perhaps Jesus himself actually had a child. If Jesus had a child, then logically his mythological equivalent should have one too—hence Superman Jr. Of course, Jesus himself is also a myth, whether he was real or not—sort of like Robin Hood. So what does it mean that these god-like characters are all having children? It means that we too are God! If Jesus had any offspring, then there could be millions of people in the world with a biological link to him. This could make any one us a part of God—or whatever your idea of an all-powerful energy-force happens to be. This is the message our myths are trying to convey. We are coming to the discovery that we are all God, and therefore have God's powers. Of course, anyone who's read the Bible carefully enough knows that this is already in there when it says that God made us in His own image, meaning that God made us just like Him. It also says that God is everywhere and in everything, which would include us.

So, our myths are not contradicting each other. They are simply clarifying themselves through enhancements of our familiar myths, and the message they are now sending out is that we are God. All of us. That's why there are so many movies and TV shows out recently about ordinary people with amazing superpowers. They are trying to tell us that we all have this amazing power inside of us—a power that will become more and more apparent as we evolve. From NBC's *Heroes* to USA Network's *The 4400* to the popular *X-Men* movies to M. Night Shyamalan's *Unbreakable* to dozens more. No longer is the superhero some mysterious being separated from us by a secret disguise. Even the second Spider-Man movie had the amazing web-slinger lose his mask not once but *three* times—once to his enemy, once to his lover, and once to the general public. Our God has been unmasked, and he turns out to be one of us. (Another clue, "What If God Was One of Us?" asked singer/songwriter, Joan Osborn.) No, the superhero is not going to save us—we are the superhero and are meant to save ourselves. The Messiah isn't coming—*we* are the Messiah!

The idea of humanity having a savior has been at the forefront of our collective mythology for millennia, but now, this theme is being clarified with the notion that we must all work together to achieve our own salvation. In fact, Nickleback's song "Hero," featured in the first Spider-Man film, illustrated this theme perfectly: "And they say that a hero can save us. I'm not gonna stand here and wait." No need to wait for the hero (Messiah) because we can all be heroes. Interestingly, because so many people are used to the "hero as savior" myth, many misinterpreted these lyrics as: "And they say that a hero can save us. I'm not gonna stand *in the way*." Someone really ought to conduct a psychological study by playing this song to a group of people to see if those who are waiting for a Messiah are more likely to interpret the lyrics as "I'm not gonna stand in the way," while those who believe we must save ourselves hear "I'm not gonna stand here and wait." Amazing how the mind causes us to see and hear things according to our own preconceived beliefs. And that's a big clue as to what's going on with *Lost*, but we'll get to that later.

Another movie theme song that plays off of the ordinary person as savior myth is the Wallflowers version of "Heroes," which was used in the 1998 *Godzilla* film. "We can be heroes. Just for one day," the lyrics suggest. While the song was originally recorded in the 1970s by David Bowie as a classic forbidden love story, pairing the remake with the new *Godzilla* enabled it to take on a different meaning: that of everyone joining together to help save the world. Of course, it is entirely possible that Bowie was tapping into this meaning with his original version as well. It should come as no surprise to anyone that Bowie has always been more than slightly ahead of his time.

So if the media myths are telling us that we are our own last hope for survival, how exactly are we to go about saving ourselves? It's one thing to tell us what we have to do, but it's another thing entirely to tell us *how*. Luckily, once again, media myths provide an answer. According to many current movies, books, and TV shows, each of us has a unique role to play in bringing about the world's salvation. Each of us has a special gift, something we're good at … something we feel deep down … something that's waiting to be called upon so that it might lead us to our destiny—a superpower, if you will. This theme is yet another mythical message of the superpower shows and movies previously mentioned, especially *Heroes*. And it's showing up in other places as well.

If you're interested to know what your gift might be and how you might use it for the betterment of humanity, you just might want to look to M. Night Shyamalan's *Lady in the Water* for inspiration. The film's universal message—that each of us plays an important role in the destiny of our world—is illustrated using the microcosm of a Philadelphia apartment complex to play out the story. Incidentally, the idea of using an isolated location to represent the world at large is common to many myths. Here, Shyamalan expertly uses the apartment complex with its Asian, African-American, Latino, Indian, and Caucasian residents to serve as an analogy for our multicultural planet.

Personally, I feel that Mr. Shyamalan is the severely under-appreciated, leading modern-day shaman of America. He is someone who can take the messages of the collective unconsciousness and translate it for the masses. Obviously, he's touched many people, since his movies continue to do well despite the fact that reviewers have hated every one of them that's been released since *The Sixth Sense*. Regardless of the critics, I will defend my stance on M. Night's position as America's head shaman, simply by pointing out that this title is hidden in his name—M. Night SH(y)AM(al)AN. There are no coincidences, as any *Lost* fan can tell you. Speaking of which, what does any of this have to do with *Lost*? I was just getting to that.

Lost Is a Microcosm of the Universe

So far, I've sort of been making you go through a lot of wax on/wax-off, paint the fence, and sand the floor, without really explaining how any of this relates to *Lost*. Well, let's review some of the points I've made so far, and I think you'll be able to see where I'm going with all this.

- *Lost* is more than just a show. It's a microcosm of the real world. How the series ends isn't nearly as important as what it is teaching us in its weekly episodes.

- Usually, a good myth will disguise the truth it's based upon. It does this because the rational, conscious mind isn't what's aware of this truth—the *unconscious* mind is. So, in order to reach that part of you, the story must speak a language that can sneak past your logical, thinking brain and head down to the cellar of your deeper consciousness.

- *Lost* is based on the same myth as *The Matrix (which is also the same myth as The Wizard of Oz, Alice in Wonderland, etc.).* These myths illustrate that life is an illusion that requires us to go on a quest to discover who we really are and that we can go home at any time simply by waking up to this truth.

- The message our myths are now sending out is that we are God. All of us.

- The superhero is not going to save us—we are the superhero and are meant to save ourselves.

- Each of us has a unique role to play in bringing about the world's salvation. Each of us has a special gift, something we're good at … something we feel deep down … something that's waiting to be called upon so that it might lead us to our destiny. (The NBC show *Heroes* perfectly illustrates this myth.)

- The idea of using an isolated location to represent the world at large is common to many myths.

In other words, the island of *Lost* is really planet Earth. All the people on *Lost* represent all of us, and all the things that happen on *Lost* are the things that really happen on our world, but our world is just too big for us to notice. Just as the island seems alive, sometimes our world seems alive, leading us to chance encounters and events that almost seem scripted. And whenever we follow the clues, or listen to the whispers, or act in spite of our fears, we usually are rewarded by getting one step closer to our destinies—one step closer to getting off our illusionary island.

According to the myth of *Lost,* the world we live in is an illusion—a materialistic wonderland created to help us experience ourselves as individuals. Why should we have to experience ourselves this way? Because we're really all one. We're all God, the light, energy—whatever you want to call it. We're not actually individuals at all. You are *everybody*! Just to clarify, I'm going to expand upon this "world as illusion" concept a bit further, using our familiar notion of God to explain why our universe might have been created to begin with.

Let's pretend that you are the almighty biblical God. You created yourself, and you know exactly how you did this. In fact, you know everything, you *are* everything, and you are all-powerful. There is nothing you can't do. There is nothing that isn't you. And there is nothing you do not know. Except for one thing—you don't know what it's like to *not* be you. Of course, not knowing something is impossible! You're God—the all-seeing, all-knowing, almighty God! You know all there is to know, but because of this you don't. You don't know what it's like to not be you, since you are all there is. Ladies and gentlemen, we have a paradox. Instantly, there's a big bang, and an illusionary world is created which is made up of God split into all these different segments. Now, all these segments are still a part of God, but they don't know that, enabling God to learn what it's like to not be Himself. In other words, God is experiencing Himself without realizing He's doing this. The paradox is solved, and our universe is created. We are all God experiencing Himself. We are all the mind of God. That is why we're here. All we're trying to do now is remember this so we can all consciously become God once more and the process can start all over again. This is the truth that so many stories have been plugging into for thousands of years. And this is the hidden truth of *Lost*.

Just for the record, when I speak of God in this book, I'm not trying to force any religious belief on anyone. I'm just using the concept of God because it is one everyone has heard of. If it makes you uncomfortable, please feel free to substitute God with Buddha, The Light, cosmic consciousness, universal energy, The Supreme Being, or Eric Clapton. The point is I'm using God because He's the being that the most people believe in, so it's just easier. If you don't believe in God, you probably at least believe in energy, so use that. They're the same thing anyway—invisible, omnipresent, can't be created or destroyed, all-powerful, can make toast, etc.

Getting back to *Lost*, you've probably noticed that all the characters on the island have ... hmm, how to put this delicately ... issues. Issues that have drastically affected their lives (or lack thereof) before the crash. Now, according to the *Lost* myth, life is an illusion that requires us to overcome our fears and bad habits so we can grow as human beings. And once we've recognized this truth or conquered our challenges, we can leave. How has *Lost* shown us this? I'll use a secondary character from the first season as an example—Leslie Arzt.

Leslie Arzt was a high school science teacher and, because of this, was very conscious of cliques. On the island, he complained about how certain influential castaways all seemed to be a part of a popularity clique that he and most of the other survivors were not a part of. Despite this, he volunteered to join Jack, Kate, and Hurley to search for dynamite at the Black Rock with Danielle Rousseau because—as he claimed—he knew how to handle dynamite. Once the journey began to get dangerous, however—with the monster roaming around and all—Arzt chickened out and fled the group. Eventually, Arzt found the courage to return to help transport the dynamite. Moments after he handled it, the dynamite blew up, causing his demise.

Arzt, it would seem, had two main issues: not feeling accepted and lack of courage. By returning to help the group handle the dynamite, despite the many dangers, he was able to overcome both issues, and thus no longer needed to be a part of the illusionary island any longer. Similarly, when Boone got over his obsession with his stepsister, Shannon, he died—as did Shannon when she got over her many issues, which included selfishness (conquered by taking care of Walt's dog Vincent), issues with men (conquered by having a seemingly loving relationship with Sayid), and her lack of independence (conquered by going into the jungle after Vincent when he'd run off). Ana Lucia Cortez, who had repressed anger and vigilante issues, died shortly after she couldn't bring herself to kill Ben. And there are other examples as well.

The law of *Lost* is that once you conquer your demons, you're free to leave. And since the island is really an illusion, none of the characters who have died are really dead. Just as when we die in our illusionary, so-called "real" life, we don't really die if you believe in a soul. The creators of *Lost* seem to, and that's why the show is riddled with religious symbolism and meaning. Some are obvious, such as the Virgin Mary statues which held the last temptation of Charlie, and some are more subtle, such as the Hanso Foundation being an anagram for Noah's. This is particularly interesting if you relate Oceanic Flight 815 to the Biblical passage in Genesis 8:15, where God commands Noah to replenish the world after the flood. Why all the religious themes and symbolism? Is the island some kind of purgatory where the survivors are being tested to see if they'll go to heaven or hell? The creators have denied it, though there's no denying that the survivors are being tested in some way—tested to see whether they can purify their wretched souls. This is not because they're in purgatory, however. I believe there's a much more intriguing reason—a reason more befitting of a show called *Lost*.

Why Is the Show Called *Lost*?

Have you ever really stopped to think about why the show is called *Lost*? Wouldn't it have been more appropriate to call it *Marooned* or *Trapped* or *Survivor Meets X-Files*? Even calling it *Mysterious Island* or *Survival of the Fittest* would have made more sense. But no, the show is called *Lost*. This being the case, the series cannot be resolved until the survivors are found. But how? It is apparent that they cannot be rescued by ordinary means since they aren't in an ordinary place. Even if they do make it off the island, it doesn't necessarily mean they will be truly saved, as was the case with Jack in the third season finale. Therefore, the only way these lost souls could be found is if they find themselves. This is the main message of *Lost*—find yourself, and you will be free.

Considering what deep issues all the survivors on *Lost* have, there is no doubt that they are indeed lost souls. This obvious point is what originally led many people to believe that the survivors on *Lost* weren't really survivors at all but had, in fact, died and were in purgatory. As I mentioned earlier, the creators have flatly denied this theory, but what can't be denied is that this notion fits. Whatever the solution to the show ends up being, the lost soul aspect of the characters should definitely play a part in the explanation.

Another interesting fact that relates to the title of the show is that in just about every episode—if not every episode—someone, somewhere,

21

in some way, will mention the word "lost." Either someone talks about being physically lost or says they don't want to get lost. Or someone says that doing something is a "lost cause," that someone should "get lost," or that somebody is reminiscing over a "lost love" or has perhaps "lost" his mind. While this could serve as yet another clue as to the lost soul nature of the characters, I think it's just the writers having fun—the purpose probably being nothing more than a word to chug to for a *Lost* drinking game.

What hasn't been lost on most viewers is that, while watching the show, most of us are also lost, as in wondering what the hell is going on. This should be expected since, mythologically speaking, the show is really all about us. Chances are, you relate to a particular character on the show. Whether it be Jack, Kate, or, God forbid, Sawyer, you feel a particular affinity towards one of them. That's because that character is you and, therefore, embodies your issues and challenges. Personally, I relate the most to Locke—a spiritual guy in a material world. I understand his hopes, his fears, and his challenges. Who your favorite character is most likely relates to your life challenges, and watching the series each week could subliminally (or even consciously) teach you how to deal with them, thereby enabling you to no longer be lost after all.

Archetypes—Why You Probably Know a Jack, Hurley, and Kate

I f you think about it, just about everyone you've ever met tends to fit into a particular personality type. While you may have your own terms for these various personalities, their characteristics are usually the same. Surely, you know someone who's a go-getter—an ambitious A-type personality who usually does well in business, but might need some help with relationships. Then there's the drama queen—an emotional, reactive person who always makes a big deal out of everything and whose life seems like something out of a soap opera. Close cousins to go-getters are busy-workers—people who fill their time up with meaningless activities so they don't really have to deal with their lives. Then there's the prince or princess—the spoiled brat who's used to getting his or her way. You probably also know someone who fits the mold of a loser—someone who just can't seem to get a break and is always having shit happen to them. And also a winner—a lucky stiff who could slip on shit but end up falling into piles of cash. And surely you know at least a couple of health-nuts—pill-popping health freaks who work out regularly, avoid anything unhealthy, and are all always spouting off about everything that's bad for you. Similarly, there's the addict—someone addicted to anything ranging from drugs, alcohol, or caffeine to gambling, TV, sex, or just being miserable. There's also the nerd, the jock, the funny fat guy, the poor-me, the all-around nice-guy,

23

the loner, the sponger, the free-spirit, the eternal kid, the sidekick, the bully, the baby, and the totally hot babe. There are many more, but you get the point.

All of these personalities are what is known as archetypes. Archetypes are perfect examples of a type or group. They are prototypes or models from which copies are based. In Jungian psychology, archetypes are unconscious ideas, patterns of thought, personalities, or themes that we all have had in our collective psyches since birth and that influence our art, our stories, and even our dreams.[5] These archetypes will usually show up as certain basic symbols or images that we consciously or unconsciously recognize. For example, water often represents love or emotion—hence the cliché of the reunited couple kissing in the rain.

While *Lost* uses many symbolic archetypes as vehicles for foreshadowing or to provide clues, the archetypes it relies on the most deal with its characters. It's no accident the writers have utilized a few dozen repeating characters, each with his or her own unique gifts, flaws, and quirks. With such a large variety of personalities on the show, every viewer has at least one that they can relate to.

Nearly all stories, and just about every story with mythological themes, use characters based on classic archetypes. While there are many of these archetypes, most stories tend to focus on about six. Known by a plethora of different names as coined by Carl Jung, Joseph Campbell, and others, for our purposes, let's call them the hero, the villain, the damsel in distress, the wise old man or wizard, the maverick, and the trickster. The hero is the man or woman who must embark on a journey that is of some great personal importance or great importance to the world. The villain is the character who tries to prevent the hero from succeeding, usually for his or her own selfish gain. The damsel in distress is someone, something, or some way of life that needs to be saved by the hero. The wise old man or wizard is the mentor who serves to guide the hero on his journey. The maverick is the loner—the character who does what's good for himself and doesn't seem to have any loyalties to either the hero or the villain, but usually winds up going through a transformation and helping the hero in the end. The trickster is a person, animal, or creature that always seems to be getting into some kind of mischief and often provides the comic relief of the story.

While there's a number of differing viewpoints about the names and character details, these six basic archetypes are found in most mythological stories. In *Star Wars,* Luke is obviously the hero; Vader, the villain; Princess Leia, the damsel in distress; Obi-Wahn, the wizard; Han Solo the maverick; and the droids are the tricksters. Sometimes, characters take on multiple roles. For example, in *The Wizard of Oz,* Dorothy is both the hero and the damsel in distress. This dual-role was created possibly as a reflection of the growing women's liberation movement of the late nineteenth century when the book was written. Here was a woman who was learning to fend for herself. This theme also played very well into the movie version, which was released at the time of the Great Depression. Perhaps one of the reasons for the film's success was because it sent the message that those who were distressed could, in fact, fend for themselves and succeed. Like Dorothy, Princess Leia also presented a timely twist on the damsel in distress archetype, being the tough broad that she was. There's no doubt that her character was influenced by the growing feminist movement of the sixties and seventies. She is the seventies answer to the damsel in distress—being rescued by Luke and Han, not being particularly appreciative of that rescue, and then turning around and helping to rescue them. Just as myths adapt to reflect ideologies of the period in which they are created, so too do the archetypal characters in those myths. Which brings us to *Lost.*

As the creators themselves have admitted, *Lost* is quite similar in a lot of respects to *The Wizard of Oz.* While the identities of which characters represent each archetype is up for interpretation, I would argue that Kate is a perfect Dorothy, as she has run away from home and always seems to be running from something. John Locke is the Scarecrow since he's always being fooled (by his father, the undercover policeman, the phone-sex operator, and Ben) and was wrong about not pressing the button. He's also been wobbly on his feet on several occasions. Sawyer is the Tin Man since, after screwing over all the ladies of his life, he surely doesn't have a heart. Hurley is the Cowardly Lion due to his fear of "bad luck," fear of the numbers, fear of being without food, and his obvious fear of having a life since he always spent his in front of the TV.

As for Jack—Jack is Toto. He's very fond of Kate, is very reactive, makes his decisions based on pure animal instinct, and often helps the rest of the gang get out of trouble. Let's not forget it was Toto who not only escaped from the witch to notify the others when Dorothy was captured but also discovered the wizard behind the curtain.

Who are the witches in *Lost*? While not as obvious, I think the Wicked Witch of the East is Edward Mars—the officer who was transporting Kate back to the states. After all, he died shortly after Kate arrived at the lost island of Oz, just as the Wicked Witch of the East did when Dorothy's house fell on her. The other possibility for the witch could be the guy with the red shoes who had the scaffolding collapse on him in the Desmond life-flashing episode, "Flashes Before Your Eyes." Just like the Wicked Witch of the East, the man is crushed with only his red-shoed feet sticking out from under the wreckage. The closest fit to the Wicked Witch of the West seems to be the monster. It comes and goes in a cloud of smoke. It torments the *Lost* survivors, and it has especially tormented Locke—just as the Wicked Witch of the West tormented the Scarecrow.

Finally, we come to the wizard. Like the Wicked Witch of the East, this role is shared by two characters. First there is Jacob, the mysterious, shadowy figure with magical powers that the writers *want* us to think is the wizard since he is first seen in the episode titled, "The Man Behind the Curtain." The other candidate for the wizard is Ben Linus. Ben is the man who's really manipulating the action and who originally claimed to have arrived on the island via balloon, just as the wizard had done in Oz. Ben's alias, Henry Gale, which he used after being captured by the Losties, provides another connection to *The Wizard of Oz*. "Gale" is Dorothy's last name, and Henry Gale was her Uncle. Interestingly, a "gale" is also a strong wind—a wind that could blow the wizard's balloon off course or pick up Dorothy's house and drop it in Munchkin Land. So *The Wizard of Oz* has its own interesting clues as well—all classic stories do. That's what makes them classics—they're in tune with our collective unconsciousness.

My point in making all these archetypal analogies is to demonstrate that great mythic stories like *Lost* all have characters that fit certain molds and, therefore, have actions that can be predicted based upon what role they are meant to serve in the story. For example, Jack is obviously the main hero of the series—hence his last name, Shephard. He is the leader of the flock. Like most heroes, he's not without his flaws. His main one is that he needs to constantly "fix things," as his ex-wife so succinctly put it. Of course, Jack fixes anything and everything except the one thing he truly needs to fix—himself. Despite outward appearances to the contrary, Jack suffers from low self-esteem—most likely the result of not only having a very successful father, but an alcoholic one who probably bombarded Jack with verbal, and possibly physical, abuse when he was growing up. To deal with this pain, Jack fixes things. Like Shakespeare's Lady Macbeth, who tried to ease her anxiety by "cleaning" the imaginary blood off her hands, Jack tries to clean up everything around him to feel self-worth in his own life. Jack's challenge is to come to terms with his faults, get over his ex-wife, and learn to love again. Most likely, the character with the greatest potential to teach him all this is the one he begins to have a meaningful relationship with. Since Kate is really in no position to teach Jack anything, it makes sense that his star-crossed lover would, in fact, be Juliet.

The other main hero of *Lost* is none other than Locke. Mythically speaking, Locke and Jack are really two sides of the same person—which explains why they both have the same first name—John (for which, of course, Jack is a nickname). Jack is the logical man of science, while Locke is the man of faith. Both of them are incomplete in and of themselves. What they each need is a piece of the other in order to overcome their issues, similar to how the black-and-white halves of a yin-yang each contain a small piece of the opposite side. Locke's main issue is to regain his faith—faith in himself and in humanity. John has had good reason to lose his faith. He's been deceived by his biological father, who befriended him only to con him out of his kidney. His biological mother has also deceived him by leading him to his dad, knowing full well that his dad's intentions weren't pure. Later, Locke is fooled by a young hitchhiker he takes under his wing who turns out to be an undercover police officer intent on busting Locke's pot-growing "family." Locke is also let down by a phone-sex operator who he thought was having real feelings for him. He's also been through a multitude of failed jobs and at least one failed relationship, and he has a total dickhead of a boss. If this weren't enough, his own father pushed him out of a window, causing him to become a paraplegic. Is it any wonder that Locke has lost his way? Of course, the truth is that whatever doesn't kill us will only make us stronger. This may be why Locke is one of the strongest and most independent characters on the island.

Nearly at the onset of *Lost*, Locke renews his faith after regaining use of his legs. Problem is, however, Locke's lesson is to learn to use faith as a guide, not a crutch. It should serve to complement his life, not control it. Early on, Locke began to put too much faith in the wisdom of the island while not having enough confidence in himself. Fortunately, just like the universe, the island has a way of shaping the beliefs of its inhabitants and guiding them in the direction they need to go.

For Locke, this involves following the island's signs to a small drug smuggler's plane that is perched on the edge of a cliff. With his legs giving out, Locke has his young apprentice, Boone, climb up to investigate—a request that leads to Boone's death when the plane falls while he is still inside. Guilt-ridden and confused, Locke visits the sealed entrance to an underground hatch he has discovered and begins to pound on it, asking the island where he has gone wrong. At that moment, a light from within the hatch shines upwards through its only window, and Locke takes this as a sign that he is still on the right track. That is, until he learns that it is not a sign at all, but just Desmond turning the light on. This universal test proves too much to bear and, instead of learning to believe in himself more than the outside world, Locke does a complete 180 and loses his faith all together. As a result, Locke refrains from inserting the numeric code and pressing the button on the computer inside the hatch—an act he initially felt he was meant to do. When pressing the button turns out to be important after all, Locke comes to realize that he was wrong for losing his faith. He then builds a sweat lodge where he can be purified and learn of the next task the island requires of him. He emerges ready to redeem himself and does so in typical hero fashion, rescuing Mr. Echo from the cave of the ferocious dragon ... uh, I mean the polar bear. After succeeding, Locke is once again on track to his destiny, his faith restored. What is his destiny? To come to terms with his handicap and let go of the anger he feels toward his father. This is the only way Locke can ever find happiness.

John Locke is also the name of the seventeenth-century English philosopher who coined the term "Tabula Rasa" or "blank slate." According to Tabula Rasa (which is actually the title of one of the *Lost* episodes), mankind is born inherently pure, or blank, and people gain their thoughts, prejudices, and beliefs from their experiences within society. The island in *Lost* presents all the characters with an opportunity to start again with a blank slate—to erase their biases and baggage and start fresh. While this is true for all the characters, it is particularly true for Locke, who has lost his way based on all the crap he's had to trudge through. Something tells me he's going to come out on the other side better and stronger than he ever was before, even if he winds up still confined to a wheelchair, which, I'm fairly certain, he will be.

Like Dorothy and Princess Leia, Katherine "Kate" Austen puts an updated twist on the damsel in distress archetype by being a tomboy who can fend for herself. She fulfills the damsel in distress role by being feminine, relatively good-hearted, good-looking, and by often getting into jams from which she needs to be rescued (such as when she's held at gunpoint by the Others or when Jack switches her backpack so she's not carrying any of the unstable dynamite). While the role of the damsel is mostly to inspire the hero to greatness, she also has her own issues to resolve—namely, her refusal to play nice with authority figures. Basically, she's a rebel without a cause who needs to either find a reason to assimilate into society or find a good cause. Despite her obvious good looks, or perhaps because of them, Kate hates all things feminine, viewing them as weak and beneath her. She wishes to be viewed as just one of the guys and is insulted whenever this is not the case. Kate needs to learn that, sometimes, the stronger, more challenging thing to do is to obey the rules, not break them. Her good heart and wild side are what cause her to be torn between two very different lovers. Like Princess Leia, however, Kate's main love interest will most likely *not* end up being the hero of the story, but the maverick—Sawyer. But she will not fully fall for him until he begins to undergo a change. At that point, the most logical step for her would be to bear his child. Having a baby would be great for Kate because it would put her in touch with her feminine side, teach her to have a lasting relationship with someone who needs her, and give her a reason to stop running and settle down.

A modern-day warrior with a mean, mean stride, James "Sawyer" Ford answers to nobody but himself—at least, that's the part he plays in the world. It's no wonder that the only person he seems to get along with on the island is Kate, who's cut from the same cloth. Unlike most egotistical, selfish characters, Sawyer knows that he's bad and for that reason believes that he doesn't deserve love. This is why he insists, subconsciously or not, on treating everyone like shit—including himself. He has built a fortress around his heart that none can penetrate—that is, until the Others get their hands on him. Being that Ben Linus is the wizard of the *Lost* myth, it is only natural that he tries to give Sawyer—our Tin Man—the heart that he so desperately needs, if only by making him think that he suddenly has one that needs nurturing. When Ben pretends to put a pacemaker in Sawyer that will explode if he becomes too angry, he begins to break down the ice wall around Sawyer's heart. The method works, as revealed when Sawyer tries to convince Kate to save herself and leave him behind after she manages to escape from her cage. This is not particularly characteristic of a man who's only interested in himself.

A typical scenario for a classic maverick character like Sawyer would be for him to finally let himself be vulnerable and fall in love, only to die in the arms of the one who melted his heart. I can totally see Sawyer meeting his demise by sacrificing himself to save Kate. This would be in line with his archetypal character and would provide an acceptable, albeit tear-jerking, way for him to bite the bullet. If the creators are on top of their myth game, this may be how Sawyer meets his end on the island. Another acceptable ending would have the reverse happening—Kate sacrificing herself to save Sawyer. Either scenario satisfies the myth because both involve the characters going through a dramatic change and, therefore, having no further purpose in the story. Being that the creators of *Lost* like to shake things up a bit, this Kate-sacrificing scenario may be the one they choose. Unless, of course, they're concerned about losing some of the testosterone-driven male audience members whose worship of the über-hot Kate is their main reason for watching the series. Judging from the third season flash-forward finale scene in which Kate is featured, she seems relatively safe. Still, that scene does not necessarily guarantee that Kate won't get back with Sawyer since he may get off the island, or she may return.

Although he comes off as the villain, the main wizard or guru of the *Lost* story is none other than Benjamin Linus. Like most wizards, he is known by many names—Henry Gale, Ben, The Other (formerly known as Him), etc. He is also obviously very smart and experienced, and he seems to know exactly what is going on, though the hero does not. This explains why the hero treats him like the bad guy. Having the wizard masked as a different archetypal character is not unprecedented in mythology by any means. When we first meet Yoda in *The Empire Strikes Back*, he is a trickster—messing with R2-D2 and trying to steal food. In *The Wizard of Oz*, the wizard first comes across as a frightfully powerful villain, commanding Dorothy and the gang to face their worst fear—the Wicked Witch. This "wizard as villain" theme is actually pretty common. In fact, you'll find it in just about any story where two enemies are placed in a problematic situation and must work together to get out of it, overcoming their differences.

Regardless of the metaphorical mask he wears, the wizard always enables the hero to grow through the challenges he or she throws at him. This means that in spite of how things may appear, Ben is actually trying to help Jack and the gang with the challenges he puts them through. So perhaps Ben is indeed one of the good guys as he has always claimed—though we probably won't realize this until we see him for who he truly is when he's revealed from behind the curtain. These points also apply to the secondary wizard, Jacob. Once we find out who Jacob is, we'll probably learn that he too is one of the good guys trying to help the hero and his friends on their journey to redemption.

The trickster or "Gleek" as I call it (named after the troublesome blue space monkey from the old *Superfriends* cartoons) in *Lost* is Hurley. Hurley is the big, lovable, yet troubled loser who usually provides comic relief during the tense moments of the show. Tricksters often have an uncanny ability of stumbling upon important clues or inadvertently helping the hero on his journey. (Finding the Dharma van and using it to rescue Jin, Sayid, and Bernard is a perfect example.) Because they are seemingly innocent, secondary characters, tricksters are sometimes used to hide important plot points since they're usually the last characters we expect to play important roles. This was the case with Kevin Spacey's gimp-like character in *The Usual Suspects*.

In *Lost*, Hurley is the only character to have consciously experienced the ubiquitous set of numbers in his life before noticing them on the island. (The numbers 4, 8, 15, 16, 23, and 42 mysteriously show up frequently on the island and in flashbacks.) He is also the only character to have been able to have a conversation with a character on the island who supposedly doesn't exist—Dave, his imaginary friend, who seemed to think that Hurley wasn't really on the island at all. Using Dave as a vehicle to express this possibility was the creators' way of having us doubt a likely solution to the show by casually putting it right in front of our noses. Very rarely in myths do ghosts or presumably imaginary characters show up speaking anything but the truth—especially when they show up out of thin air and disappear as quickly. Like Hamlet's father's ghost, Cinderella's fairy godmother, Scrooge's former partner Jacob Marley, or Locke's visions of Boone and Walt, these characters provide information that mortal characters can't know. Such is most likely the case with Dave, but we'll explore more about that later. For now, let's just say that Hurley may end up being the key to solving the *Lost* mystery.

So, we've got our hero—or in this case, heroes—and we've got our damsel in distress, our maverick, wizards, and trickster. All right, so who's the villain? Early on, it might seem like the Others, but despite their strange methods, they do seem to be helping the *Lost* gang in the long run. This is not typical for a villain. The villain is supposed to present the obstacles for the main characters. This may help them to grow, but unlike the wizard's challenges, helping the main characters is not the villain's intent. Well, what are the castaways ultimately trying to do? Get off the island. So it would seem that the island itself is actually the villain. Sort of. The island is like the illusionary physical world we all live in. A world where we become so preoccupied with survival that we forget our souls and, therefore, our destiny.

It's no wonder that so many people thought that the *Lost* gang had died on that plane crash and were now in purgatory because that myth matches exactly with what the island represents—the hellish struggles of life. However, this is just looking at one side of the equation. Life may be hell, but, if it is, it's only that way to help us become stronger. You can't get stronger by tanning on a beach all day long, as Shannon would do. No, you get stronger by working out. There's a reason it's called *working* out—if you're doing it right, it's hard work. When you stress a muscle, it grows. Similarly, when you challenge yourself in life, your spirit grows. This is the reason why Locke is one of the strongest characters on the show. He's been through the most crap. Life is meant to challenge us so that we can grow. And because the island is a metaphor for the way life really works, its purpose is also to challenge the characters so they can grow. This is what the villain typically does, albeit unintentionally.

At its foundation, the villain represents our archetype of Satan. And contrary to what current religious dogma might suggest, Satan is actually a blessing in disguise because without the temptation, without the challenges of life, there would be nothing to overcome—nothing to do. Life would be easy, and we'd all get fat and lazy and ripe for an alien invasion to give us Earthlings a severe ass whooping, turn us into slaves, and then harvest us for food. So, it's a good thing that Satan's around. If it weren't for Satan—or the material world, which is basically what Satan is—we'd all be in heaven. And if heaven is so great, we wouldn't have all left it for this place.

So the island represents an aspect of the villain as it prevents the characters from leaving and getting on with their lives. But it also represents an aspect of the wizard, providing clues and challenges to help the main characters shed their weaknesses. The island is a mentor, guiding the gang to things they need to see—whether it's a cave shelter near a stream, a case full of guns, a hatch full of food, or a ship full of dynamite. The island will always present the castaways with exactly what they need, when they need it, in order to help them on their life journeys. Again, this is how life really works. And this is what the show is trying to teach us.

Besides the island, I would argue that there is, in fact, another villain on *Lost*. It's not the polar bear, the Dharma Group, Rousseau, or even the numbers. It's the characters themselves, at least the flashback versions of who they were before arriving on the island. (Or, in Jack's case, both the flashback and flash-forward versions of himself.) These are the real villains of the show that each character must face and conquer. Some of the characters have already done this, and interestingly, whenever they do, they die. As I've noted before, this is because, once they get over their issues, there's nothing more for them to do, so they leave.

Being that the island is one-half of the villain and that the dark side of the characters is the other half, is there something on the show that can tie the two together and represent the full embodiment of the villain? Yes … it's the monster. Hence, its name—"monster." The monster is part of the island, but whenever it gets its smoky paws on one of the castaways—whether it be Locke, Mr. Eko, or whoever—it shows them their dark side so to speak. Sort of like the dark part of the forest on Dagobah that Luke had to face in *The Empire Strikes Back*. Early on in *Lost*, the monster was invisible, representing the hidden fear that lurks deep within our subconscious. Once Locke came face to face with it and overcame it, the monster began to show itself. Much like our fears, it really has no tangible form. It just creeps along, showing up during the tensest moments. As mentioned earlier, because of everything Locke's been through, it follows according to myth that he should be the first one to overcome the monster. However, once doubt began to rear its ugly head, Locke is then attacked by the monster, proving that our inner demons can resurface, even after they've seemingly been conquered. As long as Locke is still on the island, he obviously still has work to do.

The monster doesn't really show up as much as it used to because its original purpose was to keep audiences involved in the mystery of the show while that mystery was unraveling. The *Lost* creators wisely used the monster as a mysterious vehicle to draw us in. Without it, there would be no indication that this wasn't an ordinary island. The creators set up that precedent early, and because they did, the other mysteries followed right behind in the very wide path it cleared as it smashed its way through the trees.

So far, I've only pointed out the archetypes for the main characters of the show. Claire, Sun, and Penelope Widmore, much like Kate, also represent damsels in distress. And in her own warped way, Rousseau does as well. In fact, she just might be the *most* distressed damsel, since she has spent sixteen years of her life looking for her (supposedly) kidnapped daughter. Sayid, Desmond, and the late Boone, like Jack and Locke, also represent heroes. Though, in spirit form, Boone has transformed into a wizard, a role that Mr. Eko fulfilled while he was alive—hence, his long wooden staff. Besides Hurley, Charlie and Walt are also tricksters. While Walt isn't as funny as the other two, he does cause mischief. Let's not forget that Walt was the one who burned down the first boat. However, much like Boone, when Walt projects himself in a ghostly form, he is more of a wizard. As for Jin, Michael, Shannon, Ana Lucia, and Juliet, they're all mavericks like Sawyer. They march to a different drum and do things their way. This leaves Rose and Bernard. They are basically Helen and Tom Willis from *The Jeffersons*.

The *Lost* Solution—The Simple Theory That Explains the Mysteries

Now that we know who all the characters are, what their roles are in the story, and the myth that the story represents, we can figure out what the hell is going on with this show. Before I divulge my theory, however, let me preface it by saying that even if I've hit it right on the head, obviously there are many details that may or may not end up exactly as I see them. What I'm describing here is a possible solution that ties everything together according to the myth that the creators of *Lost* have tapped into. While many of my scenarios may end up *more* interesting and imaginative than what the writers come up with, many of theirs just might surpass anything I could've ever conceived. As a fan of the show who has devoted quite a lot of hours to it, my hope is that a *majority* of their ideas end up better than what I propose (while still staying true to the myth). My worst fear is that they end up pulling an *X-Files* stunt with some bizarre, convoluted ending that doesn't pull everything together with one simple solution. A simple solution is the only satisfying solution to *Lost,* and that's the reason I have faith in my theory.

Of course, not everyone will like my solution. I'm not so sure one even exists that could live up to all of the expectations fans have for the show after having invested so many hours of personal time into it. This is one reason why the creators may wind up intentionally leaving a lot of questions unanswered. My theory, however, explains nearly *everything*—nicely and neatly. While the basic theory may seem like a cop-out at first, keep reading all the details. It's not the theory itself that's so satisfying and original, but the way everything plugs into it and makes complete and total sense. Personally, I think that once *Lost*'s mysteries are revealed, the series could still get at least one or two more seasons worth of great episodes to fully explain all the details of what everything meant. And I believe this is possible even if the final piece of the puzzle ends up being in the middle of the storyline, due to character flash-forwards, as opposed to the end where most people are expecting it.

One more caveat before we begin. There may be a possibility—albeit a very small one—that you're reading this book just to learn about the myth of *Lost,* and would prefer not to peek behind the curtain to solve the show's mystery. If this is the case, you should stop reading here. I'll be discussing the solution from this point forward. Once the show has run its final episode, you can always come back to read the rest to see how close I was. You especially might want to do this if the solution the creators provide winds up to be an unfulfilling letdown. If that happens, what follows is an alternative that you may enjoy much more.

It all clicked for me shortly after watching the third season premiere. Specifically, the part where Juliet—one of the Others—is talking with the imprisoned Jack at the end of the episode. She has a notebook she is flipping through that apparently contains everything about Jack and his family—including his ex-wife. Juliet even claims to know whether Jack's ex is happy when he asks. With an almost sympathetic expression on her face, she tells him that, indeed, she is. That's when I began to put it all together. And the more I went through it, the more the pieces fit—the monster, the polar bears, the numbers, the hatch, Danielle Rousseau, the Portuguese guys at the listening station, and more. It all worked.

Just to make sure that my theory wasn't simply the hobgoblin of my eccentric mind, I decided to let a few people in on it. Most agreed that I was definitely onto something but needed to work out the details. That of course, would involve time, and time was a luxury I could not afford. The reason was because I'd been feverishly writing an ever-expanding novel about a guy who discovered that life was like an elaborate TV show—and he'd figured out the ending (eerie how much this paralleled my own *Lost* experience). Surely I didn't have time for *another* book! So I decided just to add my *Lost* theory to my notebook of ten thousand ideas I would never do anything with.

Before I could take that unfortunate step however, I remembered my letdowns with the *Star Wars* prequels and *Matrix* sequels. What if the *Lost* creators had an ending in mind that was just as unfulfilling as those sci-fi letdowns? Millions of fans would feel cheated—betrayed— by their former love, when all along a satisfying conclusion existed that no one had told them about. On the other hand, maybe the creators actually had a pretty decent ending planned. After all, they'd done a damned good job so far. Still, even with a satisfying conclusion, there was no way our endings shared all the same details. My solution could provide some alternate possibilities, intriguing twists, and additional entertainment for *Lost* fans. It would give them the chance to think "what if" before the answers were revealed. My version could simply be another possible way for the *Lost* solution to play out. Sure, I felt that it was the one the myth demanded, but I could just let the fans decide for themselves. Whether *Lost* would end with a bang or a whimper, there would definitely be value to an alternative theory. Immediately, I knew what had to be done. I had to reveal my *Lost* epiphany. My other book would have to wait.

Prior to the third season, I had three basic theories about what was going on with the show. These were:

The *Matrix/Hitchhiker's Guide to the Galaxy* Theory

According to this theory, the *Lost* castaways discover that all of planet Earth is an illusionary program controlled by a gigantic computer. This gigantic computer is the Lost Island itself. Since the island controls everything that happens on the entire planet, it is able to bring exactly the people it needs to its shores for a very specific purpose—to help the scientists who keep the computer running (the Others), and to possibly breed the next generation who will take over once The Others are too old to continue. A sub-version of this theory could have the island looking to save a small percentage of humanity as it plans to wipe out most of the world. This would fit in with the previously mentioned

Noah's ark references on the show (the Hanso Foundation being an anagram for Noah's, and Oceanic Flight 815 hinting at the Biblical passage in Genesis 8:15, where God tells Noah to rebuild civilization after the flood). Another possibility could be that the world is a ticking time bomb set to destroy (or delete) all of humanity at some point in the future. Several scientists discover this gruesome fact and set up experiments on the island hoping to somehow change the countdown in order to save us from extinction.

The *Total Recall*/Simulation Theory

This theory plays off of the very obvious fact that all the survivors of Oceanic Flight 815 have some very serious issues. Serious enough that they just might've all signed up for some kind of psychological computer simulation program in order to help them work through them all. The simulation would enable John Locke to have the adventure he's so desperately wanted. Claire could find out what it would be like to raise her baby on her own. And Michael could make up for some "lost" time with his son. Scientific experiments could also be done within this simulation much more practically than in the real world.

The Audience Is the Experiment Theory

As mentioned earlier, this theory claims that the show is called *Lost* because its sole purpose is to make the audience become lost. While audiences around the world think they're watching a show about some kind of psychological experiments being done on lost characters, in reality, a psychological experiment is being preformed on them. An experiment to see how long they'll stick with a show as it continues to get progressively more and more ridiculous: a smoky monster, tropical polar bears, ghosts, hallucinations, a four-toed giant statue, a skinny black kid who can have out-of-body experiences and seemingly make animals appear after looking at pictures of them—stuff like that. In the end, the show would have *no solution*—the joke would be on the audience. Of course, the creators would probably get death threats if this turned out to be the case, but perhaps, with a subtle tweak, they could get away with it. During the final episode the actors could come out of character, or better yet, put on some DHARMA lab coats and explain that the audience has been part of the experiment from the beginning. That, much like the survivors on the island, viewers have also begun to discover the clues that are present in their own lives, clues which are meant to guide them on *their* life journeys. The *Lost* experiment may have also helped viewers realize that we're all connected and that everything happens for a reason—even so-called coincidences. From this perspective, the audience has been an integral part of the story all along—sort of like the kid reading *The Neverending Story* in the movie by the same name. To make things even eerier, during the season finale, *Lost* could feature multiple shots of TV viewers who were supposedly being monitored in their homes while watching the show. Of course, these would really be actors, but it would all be part of the experiment. The lesson here would ultimately be that we don't really know what reality is. Even if this doesn't end up being the way *Lost* ends, this questioning of reality is actually what the myth of the show is about. This ending would just take the myth and make it literal.

So those were my theories—all based on the same illusionary myth, yet none seemed to be any more likely than any other. Once the third season began, however, I suddenly realized which of the three made the most sense. So much sense, in fact, that I knew it was right. At that moment, a deluge of connections, answers, and possibilities began flooding my brainwaves. I could even see how the creators might reveal the solution. First, there would be the cliff-hanging season finale just *before* the revelation, which might go something like this:

EXTERIOR - THE OTHERS' BARRACKS - DAY

```
Jack clutches his stomach, then, pulling his
hand away, sees that it's covered in blood.
He's been shot.


                    JACK

        Why? I ... I don't ... underst ...


Jack's eyes roll into the back of his head,
and he collapses.
```

CUT TO BLACK

INTERIOR - MYSTERIOUS LOCATION

It is pitch black. We hear what sounds like
Jack groaning. Suddenly, there's a voice.

> VOICE (OFF SCREEN)
> Relax, Jack … just relax.

> JACK (O.S.)
> Wha—where am I?

> VOICE (O.S.)
> You're safe, Jack. That's all you need to
> know for now. Just try to relax. You've just
> been through a lot.

There's a moment of silence as Jack tries to
process what's going on.

> JACK (O.S.)
> Dad?

CUT TO:

LOST GRAPHIC
MUSIC: LOST END CREDITS THEME

END OF SHOW

Now *that* would be a cool season finale. And as much as we'd like to have an explanation of that scene (Is Jack dead? Was he in purgatory after all?), we would have to wait many more episodes to get it. Because let's face it, the creators aren't going to give away everything all in one shot. The storyline for *Lost* is basically a gigantic jigsaw puzzle, with every episode being a new piece to help reveal the overall big picture. This format enables the writers to reveal little nuggets at a time while creating new mysteries—without giving the major ones away. The problem, however, is that it leaves the audience having to take a mighty big gamble. Unlike most puzzles, *Lost* didn't come with a picture on the box of what it would look like once it's complete. So there's no way of knowing whether or not we'll like the final outcome.

To make matters worse, this puzzle takes a whopping six years to put together! So the creators are asking us to invest six years of our time and energy in something that we may or may not like once it's done. The trick, then, is to not put so much weight in the final image on the box, but to focus more on the process—the enjoyment we are getting as we watch the pieces fall into place. Like most spiritual adventures, *Lost* is more about the journey itself than the destination. We are learning and growing with each piece we put in place. Once completed, the puzzle will serve to reveal how far we've come and enable us to reflect upon it. Even if we don't like the final image that's created, we should not forget how much we've enjoyed the process of getting there.

In its final episodes, *Lost* will most likely unravel its mysteries using the typical flashback and flash-forward clips we've come to rely on for answers. While it's unlikely to break this format with a string of episodes that explain everything chronologically, for clarity's sake, I've decided to do just that. For my version of the solution, I'm going to explain the whole thing—from the beginning. I mean, the *very* beginning—the early 1970s, when the whole DHARMA Initiative got started. I believe that the purpose of this initiative was to create a simulation world where doctors and scientists could study the inner workings of the mind within a highly-controlled environment. So, yes, of my three theories, the winner is … the *Total Recall*/Simulation Theory! In *Total Recall*, Arnold Schwarzenegger pays for a computer-simulated action-adventure and winds up living one in real life, or so he thinks. This theory is also similar to the movie *Eternal Sunshine of the Spotless Mind,* where Jim Carrey and Kate Winslet try to erase their relationship from each other's memories. It's also similar to *The Game* with Michael Douglas, where Douglas thinks he's become mixed up in some real-life spy adventure that turns out to be a life-changing experiment. Less known, but perhaps the most similar, is the 1999 sci-fi flick, *The Thirteenth Floor,* where a computer scientist creates a virtual universe to live out his fantasies. All four of these films share the "life as illusion" myth with *Lost.*

Perhaps you're skeptical. You may feel that it's too simple for *Lost.* Maybe—but the solution *needs* to be simple. If it gets too convoluted, it seems forced. What should be more involved is the story of how everything fits together—that's what would keep audiences coming back to the show as its solution begins to be revealed. Obviously, this isn't the only possible solution to *Lost,* but it's one where everything is explained in what I think is a very fulfilling way. Here's how:

After the imagined cliffhanger described previously (where Jack hears his father's voice in the dark), instead of revealing what happened, *Lost* returns the following season to take us back to the beginning— 1970. It is then that a group of scientists with backing from mysterious Danish billionaire, Alvar Hanso, formed a secret research project dubbed the DHARMA Initiative. The word "dharma" is Sanskrit for "cosmic order" or "natural law." The term includes moral principles that apply to everything in the universe.[6] In Hinduism and Buddhism, it is thought of as the ultimate reality and a path of conduct that one must follow in order to reach true enlightenment. In other words, it provides the way to the highest truth—one beyond what we can sense in our illusionary world.

According to *The Lost Experience* (an alternate reality game designed by the *Lost* creators to engage fans and expand the storyline), DHARMA is also an acronym that supposedly stands for the Department of Heuristics And Research on Material Applications. A "heuristic" is a rule of thumb that we use to help us take shortcuts in solving problems. They are good in that they help us save time and brain power in developing solutions. For example, if you are out in a club and spot two attractive members of the opposite sex, you may assume that the one wearing the more expensive clothes has more money than the other. You use heuristic reasoning to come to that conclusion. The downside of heuristics is that they can bring about undeveloped judgments that are often based on biased assumptions which may or may not be true. So, using our example, it is entirely possible that the hottie with the less expensive outfit has plenty of money but just doesn't feel a need to flaunt it, or that the one with the more expensive attire is flat broke due to his or her obsession with buying such pricey clothes. So while heuristics can be useful, they also can be trouble. Heuristics is also an educational method or problem-solving technique in which learning takes place through experimentation, using rules of thumb to come up with the most likely conclusion.

So, using its multiple meanings, it would seem that the "DHARMA" name is hinting at some kind of experimentation that is going on in order to help its participants find the "one true way." Of course, this concept is pretty much a given with the show and fits into any of the previously mentioned theories about what's actually happening. If anything, the name just serves as further proof that some kind of testing is indeed going on. The real question is why? A) To find the higher truth of the universe and somehow manipulate it in order to save mankind? B) To bring out proper conduct from those who have drifted from their path in order to help them save themselves? Or C), is it just to find out how long we can watch a show that continually comes up with ridiculous plot scenarios before losing our minds trying to figure out how they all fit together? I'm sticking with choice B (with a smidgeon of choice A, as I'll discuss later).

If choice B is correct, a good way for the creators of *Lost* to explain why the DHARMA Initiative was created would be through a series of (preferably chronological) flashbacks that manage to fill in all the blanks about the show. We'd soon learn that the DHARMA Initiative was formed in order to create a simulated world where scientists could perform experiments on the mind—without the usual obstacles found in the real world—in hopes of uncovering its inner mysteries. Thanks to a very generous grant from the Hanso Foundation, the project is able to get off the ground running. After years of hard work, the virtual-reality program is completed and ready for its first test subjects. These subjects would be hooked up to a computer and "placed" on a remote island within the artificially created world.

Of course, before they could find human candidates, they would first need to test the simulation on animals to make sure it would be safe. So, they gathered up some rabbits, rats, mice, monkeys, orangutans, and polar bears and proceeded to strap electrodes to their brains to see how they would react while in the simulated realm. Using the simulation, researchers could gather data on the animals using far less resources than it would take in the real world. For example, while undergoing the simulated experiments, these animals could've been actually sleeping in the zoos and aquariums where they normally lived instead of having to be brought to special testing facilities. This would save researchers from actually having to care for these animals since their normal caretakers would be able to do it from within the confines of the animals' usual habitats. Another benefit is that it's entirely possible that time in the simulation world is different than that of the real world. Several days, weeks, or even months worth of experiments could be conducted within a span of just a few hours of real-time.

Once the initial testing was deemed a success, the next logical step was to send the first human candidates—most likely researchers and scientists—into the simulation program to work with the animals directly. Initially, they probably used the cages first seen at the start of *Lost's* third season to conduct their tests, but later more sophisticated testing sites were most likely needed. It was about this time that computer programmers in the outside world began creating the various stations in order for the researchers to perform their behavior experiments on animals and, later, people. The Hydra was probably one of the first stations constructed. As we learn in season three, it was constructed as an aquarium in order to perform tests on sharks and dolphins. Once the scientists heading up the DHARMA Initiative began to focus on human behavior, they probably decided to create the other stations on an entirely separate island made for people. This way, the test subjects wouldn't stumble upon these animal experiments and inadvertently taint the results of their own. Being that these test subjects were most likely unaware that they were involved in a test, seeing a bunch of animals in cages performing behavior experiments might've made them a tad suspicious. So, the main Lost Island we have all come to know and love was born.

Despite the mysterious methods of the DHARMA Initiative, I believe that their intentions—from the very beginning—were good. For this reason, it is very likely that those heading the project sought out patients suffering from mental illness as their first human test subjects, with the hope of curing them. Perhaps this was even the original purpose of the project—to create a simulated world in order to treat those with mental and behavioral disorders. Given the experimental and secretive nature of the simulation program, another possible reason mental patients were most likely used was to prevent word of the project from getting out. Being that the project was still in its infancy, surely, the Hanso Foundation would not want to risk using volunteers from the general public should anything go awry. While the ultimate purpose of the simulated world was most likely for it to be used by everyone, testing it on just mental patients early on was probably the safest bet.

Judging from what we know about the various stations and experiments performed, it would seem that great lengths were taken in order to make the test subjects feel as though what they were doing was of utmost importance. Remember, however, that it's all a simulation, so these efforts wouldn't have taken more than some extra lines of program code in the real world. One extra section of programming code, I believe, involved the creation of an electromagnetic generator at what became the Swan station. While this generator was supposedly created in order to test the electromagnetic fluctuations located at that part of the island, I believe that it was actually created in order to add to the believability of one of the early behavioral tests. A powerful magnet can go a long way in convincing subjects that they are saving the world from a deadly nuclear reactor.

Unfortunately, this generator was so powerful it brought about what I believe was a glitch in the system—a bug that caused certain random numbers to continually reappear throughout the simulated world more frequently than they normally would. These are the very same numbers we see reappearing throughout the show—4, 8, 15, 16, 23, and 42. A flaw in the system would explain why we see them. (The universe is playing tricks on me—Microsoft Word just unexpectedly quit as I was writing this. Must be a glitch.) While this glitch seemed innocent enough, left unchecked, it had the potential to interfere with the believability of the simulated world at best, and threatened to destroy it all together at worst. Obviously, something had to be done in order to counteract it.

First, the electromagnetic generator was filled in with cement to reduce its magnetic disturbance. Then, a computer was hooked up at the Swan station that could communicate with the main computer in the outside world that ran the entire simulation program. Just as how the venom of a snake contains the antidote for its poison, and taking the hair of the dog that bit you relieves a hangover, plugging the same glitch numbers directly into the program over a specific interval (namely, a time equaling the total of all the numbers: $4 + 8 + 15 + 16 + 23 + 42 = 108$) would theoretically cure the glitch those numbers were causing. In other words, since the program felt a need to spew out these numbers more frequently than normal, they would be *purposely* created within the program to counteract this tendency. This treatment method soon led to another that was also put into effect. In order to inoculate the entire island itself from the numbers glitch, a radio tower was set up to broadcast a continuous loop of the numbers indefinitely. Presumably, these methods worked, but only in preventing the glitch from getting any worse and corrupting the entire simulation program.

One question about entering the glitch numbers into the system, a.k.a., the button-pressing method, is why require a person in the simulation to enter them in? Why not just set the computer to correct itself automatically? To discover the answer to that question, we look to the (so-called) real world. Believe it or not, something very similar to *Lost*'s button-pushing exists on many locomotives. When trains are traveling down steep inclines, an alarm goes off every thirty seconds or so which must be pressed by the engineer to ensure that he's still awake and aware. If the button isn't pushed, these trains automatically brake, preventing them from gaining momentum and going out of control. I saw a program about this on the Learning Channel. Once again, the universe gave me clues.

The same principle would apply to the button here. The creators of the simulation program had a lot vested in it running properly, so they wanted to make sure that someone was always there to watch over the process to control the glitch in case something happened. Should anyone not be there to press the button, or if it just stopped working, they would have been wise to set up a self-destruct mode—sort of an anti-virus sweep if you will. One problem with this method, however, was that it had the potential of possibly deleting everyone and everything in the simulation along with the glitch. For this reason, a fail-safe measure was created which could be initiated by someone residing within the program. This fail-safe would reboot the simulation program, knocking out the bug—kind of how rebooting your computer tends to help with any number of quirks. With rebooting, they'd still risk losing your files, but the risk would be less than doing the full anti-virus sweep. Assuming the files were not deleted, the reboot would seem instantaneous for those within the simulation—they might only hear some weird sounds and see bizarre colors, such as a purple sky, as the system reset.

This is exactly what happened when Desmond turned the key to activate the fail-safe measure at the end of season two. Doing this supposedly blew up the station, yet Desmond, Locke, and Mr. Eko somehow all survived. That's because when the simulation program came back on, only the electromagnetic generator file was deleted, so to speak. Locke, Desmond, and Mr. Eko's computer representations were saved and placed elsewhere in the program since they were all within the generator at the time it was deleted.

As the one who initiated the reboot, Desmond came back without any clothes on—almost as though he were born again. This is because he *was*—metaphorically and literally—as far as the computer was concerned. Switching on the fail-safe likely put Desmond at ground zero during the reboot, so his file probably had to be recreated from scratch. This would also explain why he was then able to seemingly see into the future. It's not that he was really seeing into the future, but his likeness had been recreated by the computer program, and therefore he was more aware of the program's details. Remember, everything that happens in the *Lost* world is part of the program, and this placed Desmond more in tune with it. What psychics are in our illusionary world, Desmond now was within the Lost Simulation. Yet I digress. Back to the chronological history of the show.

Once the computer was set up to offset the glitch at the Swan station, candidates were needed to continually push the button every 108 minutes—a perfect test for subjects to take part in. To help explain the tasks that were to be performed, an orientation film was created within the simulation and screened for the test subjects. Even though it was by now approximately 1980, and video was readily available, the orientation was shot on film. The reason was most likely because, unlike videotape, film wouldn't be affected by the magnetic energy emitting from the generator. Also around this time, another testing station—the Pearl—was created for a separate set of test subjects to view those who were pushing the button. They received an orientation as well—this time on video since there would be no magnetic interference at their station.

The test subjects in the Pearl were told to keep journals of what was going on at the Swan station, yet it wasn't the journals that were of importance, but rather the fact that they were writing them. The candidates in the Pearl, most likely, had to learn responsibility. Or, they were being studied to see how long people would continue to watch mysterious behavior and try to figure it out before questioning the point of it all and giving up. Sort of like the *Lost* viewing audience. Every time you tune into *Lost* and then run to your friends or a chatroom or podcast for information, you are, in a sense, one of the subjects in the Pearl. And if you have a computer with a camera on it, assume Big Brother is watching you, and my analogy is complete. Getting creeped out yet? As I've said, a myth is a symbolic representation of a subconscious truth—and *Lost* is a myth for the way our world really works. In fact, I am watching you right now.

Getting back to the numbers glitch, it would seem that the problem was solved. Both researchers and test subjects had connected themselves back into the simulation world to continue with their experiments, and everything was going smoothly. Incidentally, I believe that when researchers go into the simulation, they are aware of the fact that they are in a computer program, whereas the test subjects aren't. At least, that's the way it works when everything is going according to plan. Unfortunately, despite sealing up the magnetic generator, punching the numbers into the system, and broadcasting them across the island, the glitch would eventually lead to more problems beyond just the numbers randomly popping up now and then. After several years, they would be getting into the heads of the test subjects within the system— test subjects like, oh, I don't know, Leonard Simms.

Who's Leonard Simms? Remember the guy in Hurley's flashback who was playing Connect Four and continually spouting off the numbers? Most likely an early test subject in the Swan station, he probably was infected by the glitch and had to be pulled out, landing him in an institution if he wasn't there already. Sam Toomey—who Leonard mentions as the guy who first heard the numbers—was most likely Leonard's partner, entering the numbers with him into the computer at the station. Of course, this story doesn't exactly correlate with what Leonard told Hurley at the mental hospital. He'd said that he and Sam had been stationed together at a naval listening post. But remember, if Leonard was a test subject, who knows what he was led to believe upon entering the system? And who knows what he'd be led to believe after the numbers had done a number on his mind? (Just for the record, the writers may be giving us a huge hint with Leonard Simms's name: "Simms" as in the videogame *The Sims*—a game where you create scenarios with simulated people. It's just like how *Lost* works, except whereas on *Lost* the characters are unknowingly controlling their own simulation, in *The Sims*, the player has the control.)

Around the time of the Leonard Simms incident, a group of at least six researchers were working within the simulation program with the test subjects. Among these researchers, I believe, were Marvin Candle/ Mark Wickmund—the Asian narrator of the Swan orientation film— and Danielle Rousseau, the "crazy French woman." Marvin may *also* be a guy by the name of Montand, who—according to Danielle—was one of the six members of her science team and had lost his arm in the "dark territory." While narrating the Swan orientation film, Marvin looks as though he may have a prosthetic left arm. The only problem with this theory is that while the orientation film had a copyright of 1980, Danielle Rousseau probably wouldn't have arrived on the island until around 1988, since by 2004 she had supposedly been there sixteen years. Of course, Danielle never says she was *with* Mortland when he had lost his arm. Perhaps he had arrived earlier and had told her about it. Regardless, I believe both Danielle and Marvin were among the researchers while the test subjects like Leonard Simms began to get infected by the numbers glitch. And before long, it began to infect them too.

If the *Lost* world does turn out to be a simulation, it would make sense that whatever changes your mind goes through while in that simulation stay with you once you get pulled into the outside world. This may explain why Leonard Simms—who I believe had been infected by the glitch—lost his mind or made it worse if he already had issues. It may also explain why others who had been infected within the system weren't simply yanked out—doing so might've caused them severe trauma or even death, a lesson learned after what happened to Leonard.

Danielle has claimed that she was part of a six-member science expedition at sea that had heard the broadcast of the numbers and changed course in order to investigate. The scientists then got caught in a freak storm and crashed onto the island where they soon began to get sick. Fearing for her life, Danielle killed each and every member of her team and then changed the numbers broadcast to a distress signal in hopes of being rescued, but she never was. I think this is what Danielle truly believes happened. But I think her memory is very much skewed due to the glitch.

My feeling is that, at one time, Danielle was a researcher on the island. This being the case, she would have likely known about the glitch and the methods set up to counteract it, including the numbers broadcast. However, when the glitch began to contaminate her mind and (possibly) those of her science team, she may have been caused to forget that the island was an illusion, leaving her no wiser than the test subjects she was working with. If all the scientists had been contaminated by the glitch, they'd obviously all seem mad to one another. But what if only Danielle had been contaminated? If this were the case, from her perspective, the behavior of the other scientists, who all knew that they were in a simulated world, must've seemed very strange. So much so that she could've concluded that they'd all lost their minds, when, in fact, only she had. This explains why she went berserk and began taking out each of her team members, including her lover, Robert, who may have just been trying to lead her out of the system by "killing" her.

While it's possible that someone who dies in the illusionary world dies in real life, I strongly feel this isn't the case. However, I do think that once you die there, the program no longer recognizes you, and you can't get back in. So, all the scientists that Danielle "killed" on the island are likely alive and well in the real world. She, however, was stuck and quite possibly in a coma in the real world. She may have even given birth to her daughter Alex while in a coma. But I'll get to that later.

There are a lot of interesting scenarios surrounding Danielle Rousseau. It is possible that she and her team were sent into the simulation to try and cure the glitch but wound up getting infected themselves. Or maybe only she did. Maybe before getting infected, she was the one who'd set up the numbers radio broadcast to begin with. This would explain how she knew about it. If this were the case, she probably just got her memories mixed up or manipulated by the system. Perhaps, in order to get a better idea of what was causing people to get sick, Danielle and her team brought the polar bears over from the other island in order to perform tests. Once the bears got sick, they could've escaped into the wilderness. This would explain why there are crazy-assed polar bears on the main island. Whatever the details, I feel that Danielle was a researcher who fell victim to the glitch, and this caused her to forget that the island was just a simulation. Once the glitch was found to be able to get inside people's heads, it made the program completely unusable—that is, until another group of scientists and researchers provided the solution. This group would later evolve into the Others, and the solution they had was the vaccine.

If you were ever able to look closely at the labels of the vaccine, you would have seen a label which read: CR 4-81516-23 42. Yes, it's the numbers—an inoculation to the numbers virus. This is what ended up being a cure to the glitch-sickness. Once the vaccine was injected in test subjects and researchers, the psychological and behavioral experiments were able to resume. However, there was one problem— Danielle was still on the loose. Not wanting to risk her interfering with any experiments, scientists and/or computer programmers developed a security system that could track down and take out anyone who needed to be removed from the system. Think of it as a computer anti-spyware program. This security device is what we know of as the monster.

Even if my theory is completely off base, it's rather uncanny how well everything fits together, and yet I haven't even gotten to the meat and potatoes: the reason the castaways are on the island and why they had to go through a plane crash in order to get there. In the next chapter, I'm going to present a scenario and then break down each character to illustrate how each would fit into it. This should resolve most of the remaining questions about the show. And even if it doesn't, something tells me it will resolve more of the mysteries than the show creators plan on ever revealing. The reason is because a mystery is always cooler when you don't have its solution. This is why a good magician never reveals his secrets. It takes all the magic out of the trick, transforming him from magician to a simple illusionist. An illusionist is a close cousin to the charlatan, and nobody wants to be fooled. But this is exactly how we feel once we learn of the truth behind a deception—we feel like fools, and so we get angry.

About sixteen million people in the United States alone watch *Lost*. I don't know about you, but I wouldn't want sixteen million angry people on my case. Chances are, neither do the writers. So, I have a feeling that many of the solutions to the show will be kept pretty vague. Clear enough to tie together some of the mysteries, but not so clear as to be able to boil everything down to a straightforward solution that explains everything. Trust me. It ain't gonna happen. And it probably shouldn't. Because no matter what the solution, some people are going to be disappointed. That's why I feel justified in writing my version of the ending. If you don't like it, there's always hope that their version will be more fulfilling. And if you do like it, who cares what their version turns out to be? It's only a story, after all. You can have it end any way your heart—and your imagination—desires. This was how mine desired it to end. I hope it brings you as much satisfaction as it brought me. The following chapter, I believe, gives overwhelming evidence to the validity of the simulation theory by exploring why the castaways might have all been brought to the island.

How the *Lost* Gang Fits into the Equation

Ever notice how all the main crash survivors on *Lost* have direct connections to either excessive wealth or crime? They are either very rich, have a relative who's very rich, were gifted large sums of money, or are criminals. You've got Jack, who's a wealthy spinal surgeon; Locke, who has (or had) a mega-rich dad; Sun and Jin, who are loaded with Korean mafia dough; and Hurley, who won millions in the lottery. Michael's ex-wife (Walt's mom) was incredibly rich. Bernard is a well-off dentist who can afford a nice car and eat at a very fancy restaurant when he proposes to Rose. Boone—and by association Shannon—come from money, and Desmond's lover, Penelope, seems to have all the money in the world. Claire's biological father is Christian Shephard—a very wealthy chief of surgery who also happens to be Jack's father. If that isn't enough, Claire also knows a supposed psychic who has enough money to throw several thousand dollars at her, so she can afford to take a plane to America to meet her baby's future adoptive parents. What a nice guy.

Then there's Kate, Sawyer, Ana Lucia, and Mr. Eko, who all are (or were) on the run from the law. (To keep this simple, I'm going to refer to supposedly dead characters in the present tense because I believe they're all still alive outside the simulation.) Mr. Eko also has large sums of money from his illegal drug dealings. Charlie fits into several scenarios since he's a former rock star and junkie who almost married a very rich woman (Lucy Heatherton). As for Sayid, he's a traitor and war criminal in his native Iraq, not to mention a torturer of human beings. In addition, after his favors for the U.S. government, he is seemingly given lots of dough. Libby has a freaking boat—supposedly named after her by her dead husband—that she gives to Desmond for free, so she's probably loaded. And that pretty much covers all the main castaways. Interesting, isn't it?

Now, you may say that this is, after all, the magical land of television, and *Lost* is really nothing more than a glorified soap opera explaining why the characters fall into either the rich or criminal categories. Incidentally, this observation would also explain why Oceanic flight 815 had a much higher sampling of incredibly hot women (and men) than mere chance would suggest. Okay, the beautiful people of *Lost* I attribute to TV land, ratings, etc. But the fact that all the castaways have connections to money or crime, which *Lost* has gone out of its way to point out, I attribute to something else. And it's this something that explains why all of them are on the island.

When we last left our chronological explanation of the show, a group of researchers had just developed a vaccine that provided the antidote to the numbers computer glitch. These researchers, with the possible help of programmers on the outside world, also helped create the security system, known as the monster, to take someone out of the program when they became disruptive. But why go through the hassle? Why not just pull off the electrodes of the subject in the real world, disconnecting them from the program? Why? Ever see *The Matrix*? You can't just yank someone out of a computer simulation. Like anything you have mounted on your computer desktop, you need to eject it properly or risk messing up the data—in this case, the data being the subject's mind. As mentioned previously, Leonard Simms was most likely not properly removed, leaving the numbers glitch stuck in his head. However, if someone is killed from within the program, they are ejected, so to speak, and can easily be disconnected from it … alive and well. Regardless of whether this simulation explanation is the one the creators have in mind, everything does seem to be starting to come together. While I'm obviously not going to get the details exactly right, I'll now describe a scenario that could explain how and why the *Lost* gang is on the island and what they need to do to get off.

We begin this part of the explanation within a hypothetical flashback of the so-called real world of *Lost*. In other words, outside of the simulation. This is the world that we—and all the characters—believe to be real (though, according to the *Lost* myth, actually isn't real either, but let's forget that for now). Somewhere, not in Portland, the DHARMA Initiative has every reason to be incredibly happy. After two decades of testing, their computer simulation world seems to be working incredibly well, and now—thanks to the new vaccine—even its glitches are pretty much under control. After having tested the simulation on animals and then mental patients, now they are finally ready for the next step ... criminals. Naturally, the folks at DHARMA (or a competing group of scientists and researchers which I'll discuss later) are looking to make some big bucks with their amazing virtual world. Luckily for them, its uses are endless. It could be used for military training, criminal reconditioning, psychological and behavioral treatments, scientific experimentation, driving lessons, you name it.

Being that the government has the deepest pockets, it makes sense that DHARMA would have contacted them about their amazing invention. To test it out, the government may have decided to round up some volunteer prisoners with the promise of reducing their sentences. If so, DHARMA not only has to get these criminals to take to the virtual world, but also transform them into productive members of society. Since criminals are most likely smarter than mental patients, DHARMA will somehow need to bring them into the program without their wondering exactly how they've gotten there. Leonard Simms and his ilk may have just been downloaded into a testing room, without any questions asked. But these guys aren't going to fall for that. They will need some kind of an explanation as to how they arrived on an island.

Enter the disaster scenario. Begin the computer simulation with some kind of voyage that goes awry. Put the criminals on a ship or a plane and have it crash on the island. And feed them false memories as to how they got to the plane. (False, implanted memories were also used in *Blade Runner*). This way, they don't try to fight the simulation as being too unbelievable. Incredibly, the plan works, and the government continues with the program. Of course, they still want to keep the program on the down low, so they don't start shipping off prisoners by the hundreds or anything, just enough to continue with the experiments.

For this reason, DHARMA has to get some new candidates in order to turn a profit. So they begin putting out their feelers to those who could afford it—millionaires, preferably crazy millionaires. Millionaires who might want to—oh, I don't know—travel around the world in a hot air balloon like the original Henry Gale (whose "body" Sayid later finds buried underneath the crashed balloon). Perhaps the real Mr. Gale is obsessed with taking a trip around the world in a hot air balloon and signs up for the simulation to practice. Or, perhaps he is one of the first test-criminals and just thinks he is a millionaire flying a balloon that has crashed on the mysterious island (not unlike the balloon in the Jules Verne book called, of all things, *Mysterious Island*). Either way, we now have a reason for the virtual versions of criminals and millionaires, with complex fantasies or issues, to be chilling out on the same island. Of course, they cannot be left to their own devices—they must be guided. Subtle hints are dropped before them by the programmers in the outside world, and once the test subjects have made enough progress, they meet with the social workers, psychiatrists, and behavioral therapists within the program who help them on their road to recovery. This group eventually becomes the Others. (While the details of how the Others come to be is pretty much just up to the writers, I will explore a possible explanation that involves the so-called "Hostiles" later on.)

It probably takes a few rounds of scenarios before reaching the current group of castaways on the island. By this point, word has gotten around among millionaires about an amazing new treatment program that can cure problems within an illusionary world. What price would you pay to hook yourself into a computer and resolve your deep-seated issues? And perhaps the whole process, which seems to take months or even years, happens in only a few days or weeks. Every single castaway on *Lost* has a very good reason to be there. Some have issues they need resolved. Others have serious choices to make and would love an opportunity to test them out in a virtual world to see if they work. At least one just wants to fulfill a fantasy. All of them, however, have the financial means to pay for the program. If they *personally* don't, they either are directly connected with someone who does or are criminals who are involved in the government program.

Before appearing on the island, I believe that Sawyer, Ana Lucia, and possibly Mr. Eko and Kate were really in prison, and they were all a handful. After the promise of having their sentences reduced, they probably agreed to go through the experimental reconditioning program—a program which is basically *Tron* meets *A Clockwork Orange.* Incidentally, a confirmation from the show of this kind of *Clockwork Orange*-style reconditioning occurs when Kate, Sawyer, and Danielle's daughter Alex go in search of Alex's boyfriend Karl. He is eventually discovered in the mysterious Room 23, where he is undergoing some kind of brainwashing similar to that featured in *A Clockwork Orange.* Perhaps he's a juvenile delinquent being reconditioned, at the request of his parents, to have God put in his life, or, as Ben suggested, to make sure he won't have sex with Alex. Either way, *Lost* is giving us hints that the reason people are on the island is so that they will be "cured" of whatever social or mental habits they have that are deemed inappropriate by society ... or at least by Ben.

So now, in typical *Lost* fashion, let's backtrack for a bit. Let's take a quick look at every major character's personal story to see how and why he or she might be in the *Lost* world—and what might cause them to be removed, if they haven't been already.

Jack Shephard

It's no accident that immediately after the plane crash, Jack awakens in the jungle with two parallel scratches on both sides of his face. Those red scratches are the markings of an Indian Brave and are symbolic of Jack's role in the story: he's the warrior, a lonely and stubborn hero whose personal journey will free everyone the moment he learns how to free himself. This character description is reinforced by the Thai woman, Achara, who gives Jack his tattoo. She tells Jack that he is a leader, but that this makes him lonely, angry, and scared. Supposedly, the tattoo literally translates to: "He walks among us, but he is not one of us." This is Jack in a nutshell. But it's more how he sees himself than how others see him.

Most people seem to really love and respect Jack, and he has so much going for him, but he chooses instead to focus on the things that are wrong in his life. Combined with his stubbornness, this makes Jack quite obsessive. He is compelled to "fix everything," as his ex-wife so bluntly puts it. He's a take-charge guy and insists on anyone and everyone doing things as he sees fit. As a skilled and successful surgeon with an ego, he seems to have a bit of a God complex and, for this reason, believes himself omniscient. He hates being left in the dark about anything. He insists on knowing whom his ex-wife is sleeping with, and when he can't find out, he jumps to conclusions, pointing the finger at his father. He then plays God once again to allot suitable retribution.

I think Jack signed up for the experimental treatment in order to get over his ex. In a scenario similar to that of *Eternal Sunshine of the Spotless Mind,* Jack needs to learn to let go. "Is she happy?" he once asks Juliet about his ex. "Yes, she is," she says with certainty. Once Jack can learn not to be so obsessive, to be able to handle not being in control, and to let something that's broken stay broken, he'll be ready to be properly released from the island. Judging by the extra amount of work it takes to break him, I'd say he may be one of the last of the Losties to be "fixed." That is, if (as the flash-forward segment at the end of season three seems to suggest) he ever is.

Jack probably blows his chance of being cured by "fixing" Ben. It is all a test to see if Jack can let his captor stay broken. Juliet, who is assigned to Jack, tries to cheat for him. Using a video recording of herself with cue cards, she basically tells Jack what a bastard Ben is and that he should let him die. Even with her help, though, Jack still fails the test and saves Ben's life. If he feels compelled to fix even a seemingly evil prick like Ben Linus, surely he isn't ready to move on to more gray areas. Once Ben learns about what Juliet did, he realizes the experiment is tainted. So he most likely tells her that the story about his tumor is all a ruse and that she should get Jack to fix him up, and they'd try something else. This is probably the conversation behind the glass that the viewers and Jack aren't privy to. Juliet later tells Jack the gist of what has been said, but she leaves out the part about their needing to perform another test on him. For obvious reasons.

Like the other castaways, Juliet seems to be going through her own transformation. We've seen her go from an insecure wallflower in her previous life to a confident and powerful force to be reckoned with on the island. Her final test may just be to help transform Jack. Learning of this may be Jack's only hope, since the only way he will ever be able to save himself is if he learns that doing so will also save someone else.

John Locke

Mr. Locke receives a different kind of scar from the crash than Jack. His scar runs vertically from his forehead to his cheek over his right eye. Where have we seen a marking that runs down over the eye like that? On clowns. During the pilot episode, Locke demonstrated his kid-at-heart clown side by smiling to Walt with an orange peel in his mouth. What's so funny about John Locke that he's being symbolically portrayed as a clown? Well, let's remember that the clown marking is only over *one* of John's eyes—he's only half clown. He has two sides, a Dr. John and Mr. Locke, if you will.

John Locke's character is very complex. Part of him is full of self-pity and insecurity. He can't hold down a job, a relationship, or even a friend. His father used him and then tried to kill him. He's been rejected by his mother, at least two women he's fallen for, and even his pot-growing hippie friends, due to his naïve and accepting nature. And then there's his boss, who's an insulting jerk, taking stabs at what little confidence John has. It's no wonder he's bitter. On the other hand, Mr. Locke is a strong believer in fate and in the power of the universe. He's a confident, strong, independent leader. While these personalities seem completely contradictory, John Locke seems to possess them simultaneously. Within him are two sides, continually at odds with each other. Hence, the half-clown symbolism. But this doesn't explain why he's on the island. He's there for another reason.

Locke wanted an adventure. Due to his wheelchair, he isn't able to go on the rugged Australian tour he signed up for. His dream is to be able to have one anyway, to be the person he knows he really is: a confident hunter who uses the universe to figure out his destiny and help others on their paths. That's the adventure Locke signed up for, and that's the adventure he got, thanks to the Lost Simulation. Back home, he's a paraplegic who works for a box company and plays war games with his nerdy co-workers. On the island, he's a rugged champion who can stare monsters in the eye and crawl into bear caves to save a friend.

Of all the characters on the island, Locke's scenario is closest to Arnold Schwarzenegger's in *Total Recall*. In that film, Arnie signs up for a secret spy virtual adventure but gets thrown into a spy-like adventure in his real life before the program can even begin … unless, it actually *had* begun. It's the same basic scenario here. Using the refunded money from the walkabout he isn't allowed to partake in, or the dirty insurance money he got for helping his deadbeat father, Mr. Locke signs up for a program where he can experience being the person he is deep down inside—someone who is one with the universe, in touch with his destiny, and a mentor to those with problems, especially young people like Charlie, Walt, and Boone. This also means becoming someone who isn't bothered by the rejection he receives from his deceptive, estranged father—a father who'd tried to kill him and winds up crippling him.

Locke, understandably, has a lot of fear and hurt revolving around the rejection he experiences from his father. This is his main issue. In an attempt to resolve it, the Others have Locke come face to face with his father, so he can release him from his life by symbolically "killing" him. They arrange for this meeting shortly after Locke blows up the submarine—demonstrating that he has so much fear, he doesn't *want* to leave the island. Like Jack, Kate, and Sawyer at the start of the third season, Locke needs extra help, and this is when he gets it. While the man Locke sees as his father is most likely not his real dad (possibly the smoke monster or just a trick of the island), it is only the symbolic killing that matters. Locke has to let him go—severing his need for acceptance from his father, releasing the pain and anger he's caused, and allowing any lingering thoughts of him to leave his mind forever. Unfortunately, while face to face with his father, Locke finds himself unable to do the job and eventually gets Sawyer to do it instead. Using Sawyer to do his dirty work is sort of a cheat, possibly explaining why Locke doesn't die when Ben shoots him. He still has more work to do.

There have been many theories as to why Ben shot Locke toward the end of season three: he feels threatened that the fearless bald man might replace him as leader; he is jealous that Locke has heard the voice of Jacob and is in tune with the island; or he is simply an asshole. While all of these are plausible theories, I believe that they are what the writers *want* us to believe. The truth, I feel, is much more interesting. As far as Ben knows, Locke has killed his father, overcoming his major issue. Since Ben had been "freed" after killing his own jerk of a father, he "frees" Locke after Locke kills his. Ben feels that Locke has finished his journey and no longer needs to be in the simulation. Most likely, he fully expects Locke to die but leaves it up to the island (the program) to decide—why else wouldn't he just finish the job? The all-seeing program knows that Locke's journey is not yet complete. Even if Locke's disposal of his father is deemed acceptable (he does, after all, practically force Sawyer to do the job), there is still one other issue he still needs to resolve—his handicap.

While in the Lost Simulation, Locke has full use of his legs. But not so in the real world. For this reason, Locke must come to terms with not having the use of his legs and be okay with that. In fact, he has to be more than okay, because he has to realize that living a life like everyone else, despite the extra challenge of a handicap, can only make him stronger. This is most likely to become Locke's final lesson on the island. And once he learns it, he will meet his end in a puff of smoke—an end that leads him to a new beginning in the real world.

Kate Austen

Personally, I feel that of all the characters on the show, Kate has the deepest issues—and that's saying a lot among this bunch. I mean, she blew up her home with her drunken father still inside—a father who supposedly never even abused her. What gives? Kate has a marvelous way of solving her problems. Step 1: Disable person with drink (father), drugs (husband), or a bullet to the leg (boyfriend). Step 2: Run away! Run away! No doubt Kate has learned this tactic from *Monty Python And the Holy Grail*, since she too seems to be searching for something that only exists in legends—a perfect life.

Kate, Maggie, Monica, Katherine, Annie, Freckles, or whatever you wanna call her, is one screwy dame. More than a simple damsel in distress, she is a distressed damsel. What she really is, is a dude in a really hot chick's body. Let's face it—she's athletic, independent, and tough. She doesn't like being tied down (figuratively, at least), has definite intimacy issues, hates all things girly, knows how to fight and handle a gun, wants to be treated like one of the guys, and has fallen for a long-haired blonde. Incidentally, the only reason Kate has fallen for Sawyer is because she feels safe with him—not safe as in protected, but safe as in there's no way the relationship can last since Sawyer has the same intimacy issues she has. Kate feels safe because, with Sawyer, there's no chance of commitment. At least, that's what she believes.

Deep down, I think Kate is a good person. This is actually what we're led to think since we're supposed to be rooting for her. She probably just needs to learn that it's possible to be independent and strong and still be feminine—hence the reason the Others give her a lacy dress as her uniform for breaking rocks. Once Kate can adopt this attitude, learn to follow orders, and not run away from her problems, she'll be ready to leave the island simulation. As mentioned previously, caring for a baby might be one way that Kate could solve her issues, and if the "him" that she mentions at the end of the season three finale is her child, she just might make it in the outside world. Still, I think she has a long way to go on the island before she's capable of caring for herself, let alone anyone else. So if she leaves before she's completely ready, she just may have to return. That's probably a good thing since, once she leaves the show, a good portion of the testosterone-laden target audience will probably go too.

James "Sawyer" Ford

Between his many flashbacks, his numerous confrontations with the other castaways, and his time incarcerated by the Others, it's hard to remember what Sawyer was supposedly doing on a flight from Australia to begin with. Remember, Sawyer had supposedly come to Australia to assassinate the man he'd been tricked into thinking was the real Sawyer—a man indirectly responsible for killing his parents. For a con man, Sawyer sure does get easily fooled into believing that the man he's been searching for his whole life has been found and that he is someone working out of a fast-food trailer in the middle of Australia, of all places. To be honest, I'm not sure it ever really happened. I think it may have been a memory implant given to Sawyer to make him believe he had a reason to take a flight. If it did actually happen, I'd say he was arrested after the murder and thrown into an Australian prison. While there, he volunteers for the Lost Simulation experiment in order to reduce his jail time. Either way, I think Sawyer has been placed into the program by authorities in hopes of his being reconditioned.

After spending much time on the island completely unchanged, Sawyer finally begins making some real progress after getting locked up by the Others. During this one-on-one "treatment," Ben breaks through Sawyer's bad boy act with a pacemaker scheme he's devised—conning the con man into believing he's inserted a deadly pacemaker into him which will kill him if he gets too riled up. Later, he shows Sawyer that there is nowhere for him to run to since he is on a small Alcatraz-like island separate from the main island. This one-two punch combo takes the fight out of Sawyer's tough-guy persona, rendering him utterly calm and nonconfrontational. The finishing touch is his relationship with Kate. As in so many myths, beauty once again kills the beast. That is, until it resurfaces after coming face-to-face with its inner demons.

Besides being a crook, a con-man, and a really bad boyfriend, James "Sawyer" Ford has deep-seated psychological issues resulting from the trauma he experienced in his past. As a young boy, he witnesses his father kill his mother and then himself, after losing thousands of dollars to a con man by the name of Sawyer. Years later, James is about to pull a similar scam on a couple with a young boy when he realizes that he's turned into his worst enemy (similar to when Luke Skywalker chops off Darth Vader's robotic hand and then peers down at his own robotic limb). During his time as a con man, James takes on the name "Sawyer" to remind himself what a bad person he is. Since James hates Sawyer, he also hates himself, and he becomes a masochist in order to inflict the punishment he feels he so deserves. This is why Sawyer is such a dick during the first two seasons of *Lost* and why he chooses Sayid's torture over simply telling the truth about Shannon's asthma spray—that he never had it.

Even though Sawyer has a lot of issues, I think he only really needs to get over one—the grudge he has for the original Sawyer. Not only is this the same issue that Locke has, it's also involving the same man, since the original Sawyer is supposedly Locke's deadbeat dad. While this seems like an awfully big coincidence, I feel that it could easily be explained if the original Sawyer—as he appeared on the island—turned out to be a trick of the computer simulation. As stated earlier, the man Locke sees on the island is most likely not his actual father, but the smoke monster or some other illusion. Since James has no idea what the original Sawyer looked like, it would be very easy to make him believe that Locke's father is indeed the guy he's been searching for. Like Locke, all James has to do is let Sawyer die in his mind—to release the burden of his traumatic past and start life anew. With James's sharp tongue, quick wit, and excellent negotiating skills, why, there are a number of respectable jobs he could be successful at—business man, politician, stand-up comedian. Hell, he could probably even be a pretty good actor. After all, his whole life has been one big act. Look for Sawyer as a definite *Lost* spin-off character once they get off the island—*Oh, Sawyer!* Coming this fall to ABC! (Or, in the tradition of *Joanie Loves Chachi—Freckles Loves Sawyer!* I can see them on the cover of *Tigerbeat Magazine* now. Then again, they probably already are on the cover, aren't they?)

So when will James get off the island, either by rescue or "death"? If Ben broke down his macho man act, and killing the real Sawyer wiped out his demons, why hasn't he died? The real reason is that, like Locke, he's a cool character that people tune in to watch. In order to stay true to the myth, however, the story needs to create a reason for James to stay. That reason is revealed in the third season finale. Moments after Hurley saves Jin, Bernard, and Sayid by crashing the Others' party with the VW van, James finds himself face-to-face with Tom—the Other who'd shot him in the arm and kidnapped Walt. Weaponless and staring down the barrel of James's gun, Tom quickly surrenders. James, however, shoots him anyway, regressing back to his Sawyer personality, despite having strangled the man who'd created it. Whether Locke's dad is the real Sawyer is irrelevant, because James believed that he was. However, not getting the apology or the satisfaction he thought he would from killing him, Sawyer has not been able to fully release his anger. For this reason, he is now less ready to leave the island than he was before and, much like Jack, may never be fully cured.

Hugo "Hurley" Reyes

According to the simulation theory, there are actually two possible reasons to explain what Hurley's doing on the island. One is that, with all his millions from the lottery, Hurley falls into the category of the richies who bought themselves in. Despite winning the lottery, or because of it, Hurley feels like a jinx. He feels guilty about the pain and suffering he thinks he's caused the people around him, and he probably paid for the simulation program in order to learn to get over it. The other explanation is that Hurley never actually won the lottery at all, but has been in the asylum (where we saw him during his flashback) the whole time. Like Leonard Simms and Sam Toomey, Hurley could be a mental patient who is undergoing treatment in the simulation. Remember, Hurley felt like a jinx even *before* winning the lottery, thinking he'd caused a deck to collapse, which had killed two people.

Personally, I feel that Hurley just might be the key to explaining the entire *Lost* riddle. In fact, I wouldn't be surprised if the creators have already put the answer right under our noses in hopes we wouldn't notice it. While it's not part of my theory, it's entirely possible that Hurley is imagining the whole island adventure, and all the other castaways are really people from his life. Jack could be his doctor; Libby, a fellow patient (as we already know she is); Charlie, his favorite rock star; Kate, a model he idolizes on TV; and so on. While I won't be surprised if this is the case, I would actually be disappointed since this dream resolution isn't particularly original, having been done hundreds of times before (*The Wizard of Oz* probably being the most famous example).

Even though the simulation theory also allows for things not being as they seem, I think it comes from a much more original standpoint than the one man's delusion resolution. The great thing about the simulation theory is that it enables what Hurley's imaginary friend Dave told him about the island (that it's not real) to be true, but not for the reasons we would expect. Yes, nothing on the island is real, not because Hurley is imagining it, but because it's a computer simulation. As mentioned before, in most mythology, whenever a ghost of someone appears, it usually speaks the truth. Especially if the ghost is familiar to the person getting haunted—a deceased relative, former co-worker, old imaginary friend, that sort of thing. So, yes, Dave is correct that the island isn't real. He is also correct in telling Hurley that he can just kill himself in order to escape the simulation. But the delusion isn't just in Hurley's head, it's in everyone's—an interactive virtual reality game, if you will. The reason Hurley sees Dave on the island is because, being in the simulation, Hurley's mind is being explored. Everything in his subconscious is able to appear. This also explains Kate's horse, Mr. Eko's brother, and any number of other mysterious happenings on the island. The castaways' thoughts are dictating their experiences. This is a mythic truth based on the way our world really works. What *Lost* is attempting to teach us, in this case, is that our minds can create our reality. Assuming this is true, it behooves us to be in control of what we think about. As they say, "Be careful what you wish for."

Regardless of whether Hurley is in the simulation because he bought his way in or is a patient at the mental hospital, he needs to get over the same issue to get out—his belief that he is a jinx. After being indirectly responsible for Libby's death, it seems like Hurley has a ways to go. Remember, our thoughts create our realities, especially in the *Lost* world. So if Hurley missed out on finally having a really hot girlfriend, it's because he does not believe it could last. Like our universe, the island turns his thoughts into his experiences. To leave the simulation as a cured man, Hurley has to build confidence in himself and possibly even harness the power of the island, making it his bitch. In fact, he may have already done both. Taking a leap of faith that the VW van he finds on the island will start is a giant step in the right direction for Hurley. Later using that very same van to save the day is an even bigger one (and a wonderful growing moment for the character). So, Hurley's confidence issues may already be solved. His weight, however, is another issue.

While I strongly doubt that Hurley will be required to lose weight before being able to leave the simulation, it's possible that he will have to learn not to be ashamed of his weight. With his growing confidence, this could very well happen at any time. Once he has fully gained this confidence on the island, Hurley will be able to eat all the candy bars he wants without having to hide from the other castaways like he usually does. If only he knew he couldn't gain weight from any of them! As Ben's young female acquaintance Annie points out in one of his flashbacks, you can eat as many of the candy bars as you want (with presumably no negative consequences). While many viewers may have taken this to mean that there were no rules on the island, or that they were somehow magical candy bars, I believe that, since they are all in a simulation, the candy bars aren't any more real than the ones you eat in your dreams. So as long as you're not eating in your sleep, eating virtual Apollo Bars won't rot your teeth, raise your cholesterol, or pack on any more pounds. Still, using his newfound confidence, hopefully

Hurley will learn not to depend on junk food to fill up the emptiness in his life.

With his self-esteem issues probably behind him, it shouldn't take much more effort for Hurley to lick his jinx beliefs and poor eating habits. Once he does, Hurley will finally bite the big one, and I ain't talking about a giant peanut butter and mayo sandwich, though he may get to enjoy one after getting out of the simulation.

Sayid Jarrah

If the government knows about DHARMA's simulation program and is using it to try to rehabilitate prisoners and mental patients, then it most likely wants to test it on soldiers. Sayid is an ideal candidate. Since he's already pulled favors for the U.S. government against his own people, they know he can be trusted. And since he's an outsider who actually isn't in the military, word of his doings are more likely to be kept top secret.

Now that I've put this possibility out there, I'm going to side with another theory. While I think that Sayid may have learned of the simulation program from his undercover dealings with the government, I don't think the government put him in it. I think he's gone in on his own, using the money he earned from the government to pay for it. Why would he do that? To help rid himself of the tremendous guilt he's been carrying around over being not only a torturer but a traitor to his country. Sayid is responsible for the deaths of many of his countrymen. Surely, he has trouble sleeping at night. If a sweet, young blonde doesn't get his mind off of his troubles, perhaps an imaginary rescue operation might—a rescue operation where he's the good guy for once, or at least believes himself to be. There have been several rescue operations on the island since Sayid arrived, and when he isn't among those needing to be rescued, he always volunteers to be a part of them.

I think that in order to ease his conscience, Sayid needs to know that he would die for his beliefs—that he isn't a coward, but, much like Mr. Eko, he just did what he needed to do in order to survive. I'm guessing that the island will give Sayid his chance to prove his devotion, and he will do so, becoming a martyr in the process. Like many of the men he killed, Sayid will most likely die for his cause and, in doing so, will be removed from the simulation—free at last from the torment of his own guilt.

Sun-Hwa & Jin-Soo Kwon

With their connections to the Korean mafia, the Kwons have some serious won (pronounced 'wän,' the basic monetary unit of South Korea). So it's easy to see how they could've afforded the simulation program. So why are they there? Is Jin trying to curb his temper or release his guilt about his violent profession? Is Sun trying to come to terms with her inability to speak up for herself or simply trying to escape from her overprotective father? Hmm, could be, but I'd say it's more of a combination of these things. I think they're simply trying to save their marriage, especially now that a little Kwon is going to be entering the picture.

If ever there was a couple who were candidates for marriage counseling, it's Sun and Jin. But their situation is way too complex for a conventional therapist. Knowing who they are—and who they are connected to—who could possibly have the guts to give them the critique they really need? The simulation would be the perfect resolution. No matter who the father of Sun's baby *really* is, the question is whether or not Jin is capable of being the kind of father Sun would want to help raise it. Maybe Sun isn't actually pregnant in reality but wanted to test out what raising a baby with Jin would be like in the simulation world before taking that huge step in the real one. Will Jin be there for her in her time of need? Will he be able to withstand continuous crying without blowing his lid? And will Sun be able to be a good parent, despite the improper role models she had as a child? All this can be revealed, and more, in the Lost Simulation.

Charlie Pace

If the simulation theory is correct, Charlie's issue seems like a no-brainer—he's a junkie, or at least, *was* a junkie (I'm saying "was" because he kicks his habit, not because he kicks the bucket in the Lost Simulation). Obviously, he entered the simulation to rid himself of his heroin addiction. Perhaps his wealthy ex-girlfriend, Lucy Heatherton, even paid for his admission (her taking him back being contingent on his successful treatment). Or, perhaps as a former rock star, it's all part of an experimental drug-rehab center he entered. Regardless, Charlie's addiction is definitely his issue. Yet, since he's seemingly gotten over it during the first season, shouldn't he have died back then so that he could be released from the simulation? Yes (and perhaps this is why he's almost killed by Ethan), but there are at least two possible reasons why Charlie sticks around. The first is that the therapists on the outside world want to make sure he is definitely cured. Remember, he is tested by temptation several times during season two but successfully resists. The second reason is that he has more than one thing he wants to take care of within the program.

Being that Charlie's brother has begun a family, perhaps Charlie wants to see if he could handle having one too. Or perhaps Lucy wants to see if he can—without him getting intimate with anyone and having virtual sex. Enter Claire, who, with a slight tweak to this theory, might also be his girlfriend in real life, instead of Lucy. (Real life as in outside the simulation world, not real, real life. In that life, his girlfriend was—for a short time at least—Evangeline Lilly, who plays Kate. Sometimes truth is stranger than fiction.) Either way, it would seem that Charlie's objective is two-fold: to get over drugs and try his hand at a domestic existence.

Early in season three, it becomes clear that Charlie has succeeded at both these tasks. So why does he stick around until the end? Because he is a popular character, so the writers stretched out his death over the entire season. The challenge for the writers was finding a way to keep Charlie alive even though, according to the myth of the show, he is supposed to die. Their answer is a brilliant one—give Desmond the ability to see into the "future" and have him continually save Charlie from the evil clutches of fate. This stalling scenario works all season long, but by the end, it begins getting a bit tiresome, leaving Charlie with nothing much more to do.

Damon Lindelof confirmed this when he said that even though he and the other writers loved writing for Charlie, once he got over his addiction, there wasn't anywhere for the character to go. He had to die.[7] That's because, at this point, Charlie is cured and can leave the simulation. His self-sacrifice at the end of season three is even more selfless proof that he has become ready to move on. While Charlie could've easily escaped from the underwater room where Mikhail (the patch guy) had blown a hole, he seals himself inside in hopes that Desmond's dream of rescue will become a reality. Since Desmond's vision includes Charlie drowning, if he hadn't drowned, it might have upset the balance of events preventing the rescue. Charlie dies so that Claire and her baby can live, proving himself a hero worthy of true love and a family. At last, he is ready to leave the simulation world and begin his real life.

Claire Littleton

Of all the major characters on the island, Claire is the only one who doesn't have a direct connection to either riches or crime. At least, that's what I thought until we learned that the wealthy chief surgeon, Christian Shephard, was her biological father. This makes the simulation theory work even better since her having a wealthy father would explain who paid for her expensive simulation treatment. Despite working well with the theory, however, I'm still not 100 percent convinced that Christian Shephard is Claire's actual dad. My rationale fits into the whole "everybody's connected" explanation I'll get into more detail about later on. For now, though, let's just say that Claire might have a wealthy American dad she barely knows, but her memories have mixed with Jack's within the system to produce Christian. Interestingly, Claire has never once said her father's name, and, in the flashback where he was featured, Christian never told it to her. While the reason for this might be to prevent Claire and Jack from learning that they are half-siblings, perhaps the real reason is that they, in fact, aren't. Only when referencing a show like *Lost* could a sentence like the previous one ever exist.

The other interesting thing about Claire is that she's the only surviving passenger we know of who's Australian—a bit odd considering the plane was supposedly coming from Australia. (Just as a reminder, Cindy Chandler—the Aussie who's been chilling in the Others' Happy Camp with the kids—is supposedly a flight attendant, not a passenger). Knowing what avid travelers Australians are, you'd think at least half of the flight would have been made up of Australians, but no. This seems to be a pretty big hint that the castaways were not, in reality, ever on Flight 815 at all. In fact, the only way I can see that they were is if they all took it to the country or island where DHARMA's simulation facility is located. No matter how you look at it, getting involved in the program doesn't seem like something a single, middle-class, pregnant Australian girl would do. So then how *did* Claire get mixed up in it all, and why?

From her flashback, we see that Claire supposedly receives money for a flight to America (to visit a couple interested in adopting her baby) from self-proclaimed psychic Richard Malkin, who had originally insisted she raise the baby on her own. Unless Mr. Malkin foresaw the crash of the flight and Claire and her unborn baby surviving it, this scenario seems to make no sense. A more likely possibility is that the interaction is all part of Claire's created memories in the simulation, and Richard—like Libby (as I'll get to in a bit)—really works with DHARMA. Claire is probably given these memories so they won't taint her simulation experience. What most likely really happened was that she'd met Richard, and he'd told her about the simulation—a virtual program that would enable her to see if she could raise her baby alone. Very interested in such a program, Claire signed up for it. She was then given memories of Richard being insistent that she raise the baby alone because that's what she went into the simulation to learn to do. But why would Richard care, and why would he put up the money? The money most likely came from Claire's rich biological father, who may or may not have given it to Richard, so Claire wouldn't know it was coming from him. And if her father actually is Christian Shephard, perhaps he set up both Jack and Claire in there at the same time in hopes that they would not only work through their issues but get to know one another. All of this is speculation, of course, but it does seem to make sense.

Now, back to Charlie for a moment. What if Charlie's second objective in the simulation program was to see if he could handle being a family man? How could he do that if Claire's goal was to raise Aaron alone? In an odd way, Charlie does sort of experience what it would be like to raise a baby without really being a father, and Claire has more or less been raising the baby alone. Perhaps this is the best compromise to both of their objectives. Especially if they went in together as boyfriend and girlfriend to try to see which method would work better.

As mentioned earlier, there's a definite possibility that Charlie met the pregnant Claire in the outside world and committed himself to be there for her. Having been left by a man who'd made the same promise before, Claire is understandably skeptical. Once again, it's the simulation program to the rescue. Within this world, Claire gets to see what it would be like to raise her baby alone and has an option to see what it would be like to have help. Charlie gets to see what it would be like to help out with a kid without having to commit to full fatherhood. In the illusionary world of the simulation, everyone's happy.

As far as when Claire will "die" or be rescued from the island with Aaron, I expect some time during Season Four. Without Charlie around, there's not really much left for her character to do, plot-wise or myth-wise. So I'm thinking that Desmond's vision of her rescue will somehow come to pass, though hopefully in a typically twisted *Lost*-esque way.

Michael Dawson & Walter "Walt" Lloyd

If the *Lost* cast were ever to be made into talking dolls, surely one of Michael's lines would have to be, "What do you think I am ... *stupid?*" since he says it constantly. From what we've seen of him so far, Michael isn't stupid; he just does stupid things—walking into an oncoming car; going off alone after his son; accidentally killing Libby after purposely killing Ana Lucia when, with a little thinking on his part, neither really had to be killed at all; et cetera. The funny thing is though, all of Michael's stupidity somehow pays off, and he managed to be the first castaway to escape the island alive. Though whether that gamble pays off or not remains to be seen.

Walt is a lot like his dad in many ways—he's reactionary, stubborn, and always getting into trouble. If opposites attract, it's no wonder these two have found it so hard to get along—they're too much alike. The interesting thing about Walt is that we are led to believe that he may have some sort of special abilities—a certain connection to animals and an ability to project a mental image of himself through time and space.

All of this is quite fascinating, but what exactly are these two doing on Lost Island? Well, let's see. Due to his ex-wife's passing, Michael had just been reunited with his son for the first time since Walt was just a baby. That involved a difficult adjustment period to be sure. Wouldn't it be great if that adjustment period could be sped up somehow, say, with a simulation program where the father and son could get to know each other in a matter of weeks through the trials and tribulations of trying to survive on a tropical island? But alas, who would pay for such a thing? Walt's mom was loaded, so she could've left it as a stipulation in her will that they both go through the simulation in order to get money from her. Not wanting to take Walt for himself, perhaps Walt's stepdad, Brian, paid for it. Then there's the possibility that Walt's mom might actually be alive but paying for the program so Walt can get to know his real dad quickly, making up for lost time. Whatever the details of how they first get involved, both Michael and Walt most likely would have been up for the simulation, since it is supposed to make things easier. Walt may have even had the experience described to him as getting to play inside a real, live videogame.

Once the duo is in the system, however, the psychologists working within it are shocked to discover Walt's psychic abilities. Even though these abilities occur mostly in Walt's mind, in the simulation world, the mind *is* reality. So while there, his mind can make things happen within that world, explaining how he is able to project a doppelgänger of himself to Shannon. Then there are the polar bears that appear shortly after Walt sees an illustration of one in Hurley's comic book, and the bird that hits his window back home after he sees a picture of the same one. While these may be related to his powers, more likely they are just to keep us distracted from the show's bigger mysteries with yet more examples of the kinds of clues the universe gives us. The clues here would be the universe trying to tell Walt that he has powers, not that his powers are to make animals appear from thin air, though this may be a part of what he can do.

Whatever Walt's special abilities are, he doesn't seem to be aware of them. The doctors, scientists, and researchers running the simulation program most likely didn't know about them either, until he was hooked in the system. Is his power a new evolutionary state for man? A new, provable function of the mind that can be developed? There are scientific papers to be written! Awards to be won! A Nobel Prize, perhaps? It's for this reason that the Others make him take all those tests, and it's also why Ms. Klugh asks Michael if Walt had ever appeared anywhere he wasn't supposed to be. If only Michael knew that indeed his son had—in the tent of a hot, blonde chick.

So if Walt is so important, why do the doctors let him go? He's not going anywhere. Even if they do let him escape the program and then leave their laboratory, they'll still keep tabs on him. We haven't seen the last of Walt. Of course, the challenge for the show's writers is that he's a growing kid playing a character that's not supposed to be aging more than a few months. But Malcolm David Kelley looks young for his age—he's really fifteen playing a ten-year-old. Obviously, he was cast for a reason. The *Lost* creators are hoping he'll keep his baby-face looks in case they need to bring him back later on. So far, their plan does not seem to have worked. Struggling in a ditch after being shot by Ben, Locke sees Walt, who not only appears considerably older than when we last saw him (supposedly only a month or so prior), but speaks with a voice reminiscent of a crackly Peter Brady. While the show might try to write some kind of explanation into the story as to why Walt looks so much older, I don't think they will. They have enough explaining to do as it is.

Boone Carlyle & Shannon Rutherford

Boone has money, and Shannon has access to Boone's money, so both could've easily afforded the simulation program. Boone comes in hoping to get over his passionate feelings for his stepsister. Shannon probably comes in order to get more money from Boone, and in the process, to learn independence and find love. All issues are resolved, and both characters die. That's it.

What? There isn't that much more than that! Which is probably why the writers choose to kill them off early. Plus, it's just human nature to want to see rich, spoiled, good-looking people suffer. Boone isn't "the sacrifice the island demanded," as Locke says—he is the sacrifice the audience demanded. After all, watching a brother and sister have sex is kinda creepy, even if they're not blood related. *Die, incestuous stepsiblings, die!* While sort of breaking the *Star Trek* Red Shirt Rule that Boone mentions during a scene while a red shirt is slung over his shoulder, the writers strictly follow the horror movie rule: once young adults have sex—especially very immoral sex—they die. End of story.

Actually, there is another reason the island might've demanded Boone's life—because it makes Locke start banging on the hatch ... which Desmond hears ... causing him to decide not to kill himself ... if he had, no one would be around to press the button or turn the failsafe key … had this happened, the program would've shut down/island gotten destroyed … and that would have been the end of that. In other words, Boone dies so that we might enjoy *Lost* for at least four more seasons. Like I said, Boone is the sacrifice the audience demanded.

Bernard & Rose Nadler

Of all my explanations as to why the various crash survivors are on the island, I think Rose and Bernard's is my favorite. Unlike most of the other castaways, these two newlyweds don't seem to have a lot of psychological, neurotic, or interpersonal issues beyond that of most couples. They have their arguments, sure, but their relationship, albeit relatively short, does not seem to be dysfunctional. Both seem to care deeply for one another. This isn't to say that Rose and Bernie don't have any major issues; they have at least one, but it's seemingly out of their control—Rose's illness. The day Bernard proposes, Rose reveals that she has been diagnosed with a terminal form of cancer and has only about a year to live. Bernard's feelings for her are so strong, however, he insists they get married anyway. In the back of his mind, though, Bernard feels that Rose might be able to be cured.

During the honeymoon in Australia, Bernard takes Rose to see a faith healer, hoping he can purge his new wife of her illness. Unfortunately, the healer tells Rose that he can't cleanse her since the location they are in isn't "the right place." What would be the right place? Turns out to be the island. Rose, being one of the few castaways to know that John Locke is in a wheelchair on the flight, feels that the island has cured her too. For this reason, she doesn't wish to be rescued, for as long as she's on the island, she feels she will live out her years cancer-free.

So, what can this all mean? Something about the island's healing properties or longevity experiments performed by the DHARMA Initiative? Poppycock! Bernard must've heard about the simulation program and signed himself and his wife up for it. This way, like Michael and Walt, they will be able to spend quality time with one another without the constraints of reality. Since the world they have come to live in is an illusionary one, time most likely won't progress as it normally would in the outside world. Therefore, it is highly probable that Rose and Bernard will get to have more time together (at least, in their minds) than they would in the "real" world. Within the simulation, Rose isn't sick. She could be hooked up to a respirator and slowly dying in reality, but as long as she remains within the program, none of that is happening. Bernard obviously loves Rose enough to risk whatever it takes in order to spend more time with her. Perhaps they really took their honeymoon in Australia, or perhaps this is just a false memory created by the simulation to explain why they were taking a flight home from there. Either way, Bernard and Rose hooked themselves up to the program in hopes it would enable them to live out their years together—even if that meant they'd be stuck on a bizarre island with a bunch of over-the-top male egos and drama queens. If that isn't true love, I don't know what is.

Leslie Arzt

As mentioned earlier, Dr. Arzt has most likely entered the simulation in order to overcome his general fears as well as his hang-ups about being accepted by others (with a name like Leslie, it's not hard to imagine how this could've been a problem for him while growing up). By volunteering to help the most popular survivors handle dangerously old dynamite, he manages to tackle both of his issues in one shot and is therefore conveniently removed from the program when the dynamite blows him up.

While Arzt isn't rich, he is a science teacher, and this could've enabled him to have a personal connection to the DHARMA Initiative, which is presumably comprised mostly of scientists. It is highly probable that Arzt used to be a scientist, researcher, or even a physician at one time. In fact, his name, "Arzt" is German for "physician." Perhaps Arzt used to be a physician working for the DHARMA Initiative and remained connected after leaving the group. There's also the possibility he's still in DHARMA and just needed to solve some of his own issues. So, he volunteered to enter the next simulation run. Whatever the details, it seems that, unlike the other castaways, Arzt gets over his issues fairly quickly, enabling him to leave just as fast.

While the writers might seem rather callous in having Hurley tell Jack, "Dude, you got some Arzt on you," shortly after Arzt is blown to bits, knowing that Arzt is really alive and well lightens the harshness of the comment, particularly in an era when people getting blown up hits a little too close to home. The mythic message here seems to be that even when we die in a seemingly pointless way, perhaps there's a reason for it. There are no accidents—and that's a truth that encompasses even the seemingly randomness of death. Unlike the other castaways, Arzt is just a regular guy. So maybe his death, more than that of any of the other characters, is meant to serve as the most relevant message for all of us. Guess he wasn't such a minor character after all.

Ana Lucia Cortez

A tough former cop who's broken the law for revenge, Ana Lucia is the first of the castaway convicts to be "rehabilitated." While it's never revealed in her flashbacks, I'm guessing that Ana Lucia's mother (and former boss) advised her to turn herself in, in hopes of her getting a lighter sentence, and that she did. The whole trip to Australia with Jack's dad is probably a fabricated memory created by the simulation program. In the real world, Ana Lucia was probably in prison for gunning down the man who shot her while she was on duty, causing her to lose her unborn fetus. She was most likely sentenced for a number of years for this crime, but, thanks to her police connections, is able to take part in the experimental simulation-rehabilitation program—a program that will help her reduce her sentence and get over her major issue of *trigger-happyitis*.

After accidentally shooting Shannon, at first it doesn't seem as though Ana Lucia is making much progress. But it is this accident that makes her come to terms with her itchy trigger finger. Ana Lucia later proves her new aversion to killing when she refuses to put a bullet in Ben "Henry Gale" Linus's head, even after he attacks her. At last, Ana Lucia is cured, and she is "killed" by Michael shortly thereafter.

Mr. Eko

The text below comes from an e-mail I sent out to some of my *Lost* fan friends—an e-mail that I eventually used as an outline to write this book.

Mr. Eko wants a second chance at being good after his brother dies. The plane is put on the island for him to come to terms with his brother's death. He will probably die soon, if he isn't already dead.

I sent that out on Thursday, October 5, 2006 at 12:26 AM, the night *Lost* season three premiered. This was before we even knew whether or not Mr. Eko had survived the hatch explosion. Two weeks later, we learned that Mr. Eko was, in fact, alive, only to die two weeks after that. I had been right about Mr. Eko. Why did I think he was a goner? As mentioned in that e-mail blurb, I believe that Mr. Eko was put into the simulation to get over the guilt he felt over his brother Yemi's death. Had he not been involved in crime, his brother would still be alive.

Whether Mr. Eko is actually a prisoner serving time for his crimes and involved in the rehabilitation program, or using his drug money to buy his way into the computer simulation, I'm not sure, and I'm not sure it even matters. What is more important is the fact that the plane Yemi died on just happens to be on the island. If it should turn out that the Lost Island is a real place, the writers will have quite a lot of explaining to do as to why his plane just happened to have crashed there. If, however, the simulation theory is what ends up being the solution to the *Lost* mystery, this all makes perfect sense. Mr. Eko needs closure. He needs to bury his brother and say good-bye. After doing this at the end of the second season, Mr. Eko is almost ready to leave. There is just one more thing he has to do though, and that is realize that he isn't responsible for Yemi's death. That his own sacrifices in life had given his brother the fighting chance that he'd had. As Mr. Eko comes to understand—thanks in part to the simulation program/ smoke monster playing the part of Yemi—he did what he had to do. For this reason, he does not need his brother's forgiveness (during that scene when the simulated Yemi asks for it). Had Mr. Eko not grabbed the gun and killed the old man when they were kids, surely his brother would have ended up being the drug dealer instead of him and probably would have been killed anyway.

Mr. Eko did the best he could, given the cards he was dealt. After he comes to this realization, the monster disposes of him, enabling him to leave the island with a clear conscience. Moments before death, everything likely becomes clear to Mr. Eko. He probably realizes the truth about the simulation program. So when he tells Locke and company that they are all next to die, he isn't saying it menacingly. In his mind, he is telling them something hopeful—that soon, they too will solve their issues and be able to return to their real lives. I hope Mr.

Eko is there waiting for them when they do. 'Cause that's the kinda guy he is. Or at least, the kinda guy he becomes.

Desmond David Hume

When I stated that Rose and Bernard's explanation as to why they are on the island is my favorite, I meant of the Flight 815 crash survivors. Of *all* the castaways on the island, Desmond's reason for being there is far and away my favorite. Because I believe he is the only one put into the simulation program against his will. And it's all because of his love for a woman.

Before I get into that, however, let's take a look at Desmond's name. Much like the names John Locke and Danielle Rousseau (to be explained soon), Desmond David Hume's name is based on a philosopher. David Hume was a Scottish philosopher (and a friend of fellow philosopher Jean-Jacques Rousseau for a time) who believed that everything we know comes to us through our senses. That is to say, our impression of life comes to us through our mind, which may or may not be an accurate representation of reality.[8] In other words, things may not be as they seem, and what we think is real may only be a figment of our imaginations. Sound familiar? That's the basis of the whole Lost Simulation program. The castaways believe that they've survived a plane crash and are now living on a tropical island because that's what their senses are telling them, when in fact all of them are probably laying in cots with electrodes strapped to their heads at some DHARMA testing center that's not located in Portland. Since Desmond's namesake was someone who believed things may not be as they seem, it's possible that he'll be the first to discover the truth about their situation. If so, I think he'll be removed before he has a chance to tell anyone else. I can picture him excitedly running to the *Lost* gang screaming, "I've got it, my brothers! I know why we're here! It's all a sim—" Just then, the monster grabs Desmond and drags him down to its underground labyrinth. Desmond is never heard from again. In reality, he's just been ejected from the program, but no one knows that yet. Come on, admit it—this would be pretty cool. And it's about to get even better …

What we know about Desmond is that before arriving on the island, he had joined a monastery to run away from his own wedding. Later, he joined the Scottish army to run away from a second failed relationship. Before he can run away from anything else, though, he winds up in a military prison for not following orders. Then again, perhaps he disobeyed orders hoping he *would* end up in prison so he could stop running. While in prison, Desmond writes dozens of letters to the woman he'd had the second failed relationship with but still loves—Penelope Widmore. Upon Desmond's release from prison, he is met at the gate by Penelope's very wealthy father, Charles Widmore, who tells Desmond that he's intercepted every one of his letters to his daughter and offers him money to walk away from her forever. Desmond refuses, and instead, hoping to gain Charles's approval, decides to enter a sailboat race around the world that Charles sponsors. Not long after, Desmond bumps into Libby, who just happens to have an extra sailboat that belonged to her deceased husband. She says she wants Desmond to have it. Pretty convenient. Only, that's not what I believe really happened.

For reasons I'll describe in more detail during Libby's blurb, I believe she is well aware of the simulation program, either because she has been through it herself and/or because she works for the DHARMA Initiative. Either way, it's very possible that Charles Widmore (who supposedly owns a building that houses the Hanso Foundation, which funds the DHARMA Initiative) hired Libby to track down Desmond and tell him about an amazing opportunity. No, not a free boat, but an incredibly realistic simulation program that he could take part in to practice the sailboat race. This is what I believe Libby *really* tells Desmond about when they first meet. The whole boat thing is a fabricated memory given to Desmond while he is in the system to explain how he'd gotten to the island. In reality, Libby hasn't given him a boat; she has given him a tip about how to sign up for the experimental program. Desperate to win the race, Desmond will be all too eager for any edge he can get. The thing is, it is all a trap set up by Charles to get poor Desi stuck in the simulation world, never to be heard from again.

In fact, Widmore may have also pulled this same trick on the original Henry Gale—the African-American dude whom Sayid found buried underneath a hot-air balloon. Like Desmond, Gale was probably trying to make it around the world. We all know how that ends up. Another suitor for Penelope's love, perhaps? Charles probably keeps him inside the program until she has safely moved on. Since the plan has worked once, he might as well try it again. So, in trying to protect his precious daughter, Charles basically puts Desmond into a vegetative state by getting him hooked up indefinitely to the simulation program. What he doesn't count on, however, is how deeply in love his daughter actually is and the lengths she's willing to go to find out what happened to her beloved Desi-pooh.

After Desmond breaks up with Penelope, she most likely confronts her father to find out what he's said to her sensitive, unemployed boyfriend who—she thinks—has recently come to him asking for a job. While Charles probably doesn't reveal that Desmond had actually asked for his permission to marry her, he probably had no qualms with telling her how much he disapproves of her choice in Desmond. Knowing her father's cold personality, Penelope likely becomes suspicious that he'd say something to scare away her precious Desi-kins and, at that point, decides to try to win him back. That becomes difficult after he joins the army and close to impossible once he enters prison—especially with her father confiscating all of his letters. Once Desmond gets out, however, she soon learns that he is planning to enter the boat race that her father's company sponsors. Shortly thereafter, he disappears. Penelope is no dummy, and before long, she obviously figures out what her father has done and begins working to save her man.

Penelope shares her name with Odysseus's wife from Homer's *Odyssey.* In that story, Penelope remains faithful to her husband during his twenty years at war and at sea, rejecting the proposals of 108 suitors. (Interestingly, 108 is the total of the *Lost* numbers: 4 + 8 + 15 + 16 + 23 + 42 = 108.) After battling the Cyclops, sailing within earshot of the sirens' deadly song, and passing between the multi-headed Scylla monster and the Charybdis whirlpool, Odysseus returns to his native Ithaca, kicks the shit out of all the suitors, and wins back his beloved Penelope. I don't think it's an accident that the writers of *Lost* have chosen the name Penelope for Desmond's long lost love. That being the case, expect anyone standing in his way to meet an untimely demise once he gets out of the simulation program—and he *will* get out. No writer on earth can resist a good ass-whooping revenge for the love of a woman.

Now, some of you may be thinking: "But hold up, Desmond *can't* be in a simulation program because those two Portuguese-speaking dudes chilling at the listening station track down the island and call Penelope to tell her about it, and she is later able to make contact herself. Therefore, the island must really exist!"

Very often throughout *Lost*, the writers use the sweet siren song of heuristics to mess with our rational minds, causing us to make incorrect assumptions. Can the purpose of these "contact with the outside world" segments be to throw us off the trail? Assuming that the *Lost* world is a simulation, isn't there another possibility that could explain how the outside world is able to make contact with those in the simulation?

Since Penelope is Charles's daughter, she probably knows all about the simulation program, but because her dad sneaks Desmond into it, she can't just ask someone in the DHARMA Initiative where he is. So, upon learning what her father has done to her darling Desi-wesie, she immediately hires a couple of—how do you say, *computer hackers*—to get into the system to search for where he might be. That's right, those two dudes freezing their arses off in the tundra, or wherever, are hiding there for a reason—they're in the simulation program just like the *Lost* gang—but in a desolate place where its programmers—and anyone who might be in cahoots with her father—won't find them. From there, the hackers are able to locate the electromagnetic energy from the generator within the hatch, using a tracing program that they created from within. Then, they simply call Penelope using a modem connection, and voila, "We know where your boy is!" Pretty sneaky, sis.

Once Penelope has the location and a patch, she is able to link in from her home computer, explaining why she looks like she is sitting in front of one when she makes contact with Charlie at the submerged station during the end of season three. How unfortunate that the connection is lost due to the station flood before Penelope has a chance to uncover where the Losties actually are. It's even more unfortunate when we learn that Penelope had not, in fact, sent the rescue ship. So who did? I'm guessing daddy did, and a rescue isn't exactly what he has in mind. He may have sent in the ship for the same reason he may have sent in Libby—to check up on Desmond.

Since the simulation program is supposed to be helping people and not keeping them prisoner, we have to assume that Charles Widmore manages to get Desmond into the simulation without the DHARMA researchers knowing about it (remember, the Others didn't know about Desmond's boat). It is also probable that he is the one responsible for sending in Naomi, the woman who supposedly parachuted onto the island in search of Desmond. Her task is most likely to seek out Desmond and keep him from leaving. Remember, killing him would just eject him from the system, so she needs to convince him to stay. Making everyone think that they are really dead is probably the first part of her plan (hence, a possible reason she would lie about the Oceanic plane being found with no survivors). We'll hopefully find out the rest when the "rescue" crew from the boat arrives on the island during season four. My guess is that they will turn out to be a more formidable foe than the Others. The Others, after all, are really there to help the Losties. They haven't done much for Desmond, though, simply because they might not even be aware that he's there, or perhaps they have been told that he's a part of a separate project and that they shouldn't interfere.

Despite not having the help of the Others, it is still possible that the simulation program itself is trying to "fix" Desmond's issues. Perhaps Charles Widmore even set it up that way. Maybe he isn't such a bad guy after all and put Desmond in the simulation, not to keep him from Penny, but to help him become a man worthy of her. Certainly, that would be a twist worthy of *Lost*, but not one I would expect, since Charles makes such a great villain. Assuming Charles is the jerk we are led to believe that he is, another possibility is that the simulation is automatically programmed to detect and cure dysfunctional behavior. As stated earlier, Desmond always runs away from responsibility. Within the simulation, he is given the sole responsibility to "save the world" by continually pressing the button without knowing what it's really for. When he runs away from that responsibility, bringing about a leak of magnetic energy, the simulation forces him to face the repercussions of his actions by timing it to the fabricated Oceanic 815 crash. Now, he must live with the result of what he has done without being able to run away from it or the people he's hurt. He now must come face-to-face with those whose lives he seemingly destroyed—as opposed to his experience with his ex-fiancé Ruth and his ex-girlfriend Penny, both of whom he ran away from.

This insight into Desmond's flaws explains his decision back at the end of the second season to sacrifice himself to save those whose very lives he felt he ruined. He does this by turning the key to blow up the Swan station, saving the island and all its inhabitants, or at least, so he believes. Believing he will die for his "sins" is what brings about Desmond's transformation. Of course, Desmond does not die but is, instead, reborn—naked and with new Messianic abilities. Slender with long brown hair and a beard, is there any doubt who Desmond is the archetype of? Particularly since he is told that his actions would "save the world" by both his former Swan station partner Kelvin and the old lady from his flashback, Ms. Hawking (whose name is likely taken from physicist and *A Brief History of Time* author Stephen Hawking). Since the Lost Island is a microcosm of the world, in a sense, Desmond does save it when he saves the island. Afterward, he is then able to help others—like Charlie—complete their missions, making Desmond the true savior of *Lost*.

Libby (Elizabeth)

From what we know or think we know about Libby from Hurley's flashback, she has spent some time in the same mental hospital that he and Leonard Simms have been in. Perhaps Libby is also one of the early test subjects who underwent treatment in the simulation and was ultimately cured by it. If this is true, she would likely be a fan of its treatment method. This could be a reason why she may have decided to join the DHARMA Initiative, particularly since she either already was, or possibly became, a psychologist (as she told Hurley). Once with the Initiative, it's not a far leap to think she may have been contacted by Charles Widmore about doing him a favor. She probably doesn't even realize the repercussion of her actions, most likely assuming that Desmond really is going to get a sailing race simulation. Perhaps discovering the truth of what she has done gives her a mental relapse, sending her into the simulation again—this time with the Losties. Or, maybe she comes to the island because she has once again been hired by Charles, only now, her mission is to infiltrate the simulation, find Desmond, and make sure he isn't going anywhere.

Sure, this is all speculation, but it all makes sense, doesn't it? And there are many more possibilities. If Libby didn't come to the island to track down Desmond, another explanation (especially if she's a member of DHARMA) is that she disguised herself as a passenger, instead of opting to become one of the Others, to specifically help Hurley. Since they have both been in the mental hospital together, Libby may have been responsible for telling him about the program and might have went in to assist him with his issues. While unlikely, they might even be a couple in the outside world. It would be more interesting, though, if she just works for DHARMA, and Hurley pays extra for some romantic ego boosting. Once he gets his kiss, she is no longer needed. Hurley should have gone for the platinum package, which would have involved a twosome with Libby and Juliet, along with psychological counseling from both of them about his self-image and weight problem.

For whatever reason, Libby strikes me as one of the good guys who may have been unknowingly manipulated by DHARMA or Widmore. However, this just may be what the show wants us to think because Libby's motives haven't been pure from the start. If this is the case, and Libby has been knowingly doing Widmore's bidding all along, she may have been in the institution only so that she could spy on Hurley or Leonard Simms. She then may have purposely tricked Desmond to get into the simulation, and come to the island to work out more dastardly plans. This would explain why she gets shot by Michael—the island arranges it in order to protect itself. From this perspective, Libby isn't an innocent bystander who's in the wrong place at the wrong time— she is an evildoer who gets what she deserves. Say it ain't so, Libby.

Danielle Rousseau

Does it seem odd to anyone else that a very pregnant woman would have gone on a dangerous scientific expedition around the Pacific Ocean? As explained earlier, I think that Danielle's mind is stuck somewhere between reality and the simulation world. The way I see it, she was originally one of the researchers (a.k.a DHARMA) conducting experiments on patients within the simulation program when the numbers glitch began infecting her mind, causing her to forget that none of it was real. If she was the only one infected, the behavior of the other researchers must have seemed pretty odd to her! Perhaps they even told her to kill herself to escape the program. "Program! What program? Have you gone mad?" I can hear her saying in that weird, not-really-French accent of hers. If she wasn't the only one infected, one can only imagine the effects the glitch had on the other researchers. Either way, to Rousseau, all of them would seem to be very sick, requiring her to take drastic action. So, as she eventually admits to the Losties, she "killed" them all.

In Rousseau's distress signal, however, Shannon translates her as saying that, "*it* killed them all." Assuming she's even translating right, this can mean that Rousseau—at the time—had dissociated herself with the killing, projecting it onto something else, or more likely, she was planning to make up a story so she wouldn't get blamed once rescued. After being trapped on the island for sixteen years, she either came to terms with what she did or had just given up on the need to hide it from anyone.

There are obviously a number of possible scenarios involving what happened to Rousseau and the gang, but from what's been revealed up through season three, she definitely seems like a lost DHARMA researcher to me. Or at the very least, a lost test subject whose mind has been corrupted by the numbers glitch. Her name provides a slight clue. Rousseau's name is most likely taken from that of eighteenth-century philosopher Jean-Jacques Rousseau. Rousseau believed that man is basically good by nature but is corrupted by society.[9] This can be taken to mean that Danielle was good until she was either corrupted by her scientific co-workers or by the programming glitch. While the *Lost* myth allows for a number of scenarios, until we learn more about Danielle's backstory, I'll say that it is the glitch that messed her mind.

As far as Ms. Rousseau having a baby while in the simulation, again, there are a lot of possibilities. She could've given birth to her daughter, Alex, while in a coma (from being stuck in the simulation). Alex could've been born before the simulation, but Danielle's memory of her could've been changed once she was hooked in. There's also the possibility that Danielle went into the simulation with her teenage daughter to work something out with her, but then her mind became messed up from the glitch, and she got stuck there. What seems most probable is that Alex joined up with DHARMA in order to try to track down her mom and get her out of the system. That's why Alex is sort of the reluctant Other. Had she really been raised by them, as the show would have us believe, she wouldn't know anything other than the Others' way. I think a much better scenario would have Alex being raised in the real world by her mother's fellow researchers (whom her mom "killed" in the simulation). When she was young, they could've told her that her mother was dead or, more truthfully, in a coma. When she grew up enough to be let in on the truth, she probably decided to enter the simulation in hopes of getting her mother out. And that's why she's there. Alex is on a mission to find and save her mom, while her mom is on a mission to find and save her. Now that they've found each other, it really doesn't seem like there's much more for them to do. The writers will either have to create something new like they did with Charlie, or else it may be lunch time for the monster. Mmm, French food.

Juliet Burke

In many ways, Juliet is two completely different people. Before arriving on the island, she is a soft-spoken, meek wallflower with a controlling ex-husband who seems to still run her life. After arriving, she transforms into a manipulative, strong-willed, powerful woman who can easily fend for herself. There are other dichotomies as well. Is she still loyal to the Others or aligned with the Losties? Trustworthy or two-faced? Good-hearted or only looking out for herself? The only thing we know for sure about Juliet is that she's an enigma.

Despite her mysterious nature, it is with Juliet that we first see how the Others transport someone to the island—via submarine. This being the case, it would seem as though the island must be real and not a simulation after all. Closer analysis of her voyage, however, reveals quite a number of clues that prove just the opposite. For starters, why does Juliet have to be drugged for the trip? She's a grown woman and a doctor—surely, she can withstand the voyage. At the very least, her hosts could wait until she is on board before asking if she wants to take a tranquilizer. While it might seem that she is drugged so that she won't learn of the location of the island, how would she discover it anyway, being submerged in a sub? Unless ... she isn't taken to the island on a sub at all.

Mythologically speaking, being underwater (especially in the ocean) is symbolic of dreams and the subconscious. That's why the planet Neptune—named after the Roman god of the sea—represents our dreams and subconscious in astrology. So by having a submarine as the vehicle of choice to get to the island and revealing that Juliet has to be knocked out, the show implies that the only way to get to this place is through our subconscious minds. That's the real reason Juliet has to be sedated. She isn't taken to the island on a sub at all. She is rendered unconscious, taken to the facility, and hooked up like everyone else. Once in the simulation, it is easy to place her on a submarine that has just docked. Interesting that she is strapped in when she awakens, most likely because that's how she is in real life. She's even lost her voice when she first wakes up. This seems to imply that other people—like her ex-husband and now Ben—are doing her speaking for her. For any other show, that would be a stretch, but this is *Lost*. Juliet is brought to the island to do fertility experiments, as per Ben's wishes, and is told she will not be allowed to leave until she is successful. Regardless of the symbolic details, it's interesting that Juliet is not awake during her entire voyage to the island. This is obviously done for a reason.

Not a castaway and not really an Other, what exactly is Juliet doing on Lost Island? While it's possible she's there to help solve the inhabitants' fertility problems, more likely it's for the same reason as the Losties—to help her resolve her own issues. As we saw from Juliet's flashback, she is someone who lets people, like her ex-husband, walk all over her. When approached by Dr. Richard Alpert about leading a scientific team, she admits that she isn't a leader, that she is a mess. The simulation might've been just what the doctor ordered to help her improve her self-confidence, become a leader, and, in the process, develop her revolutionary fertility treatment. Another possibility is that her improved self-esteem has been just a side effect of the simulation and that her rich ex-husband paid to put her in solely for her fertility work, hoping to reap the rewards from it. This would explain why Ben is so adamant that she complete it and why he tells her she can't leave until she does—he won't get the money otherwise. If this turns out to be the case, it's probably also likely that her ex-husband was not hit by a bus, as depicted in her flashback, and that her sister has not had a baby. These are probably all tricks of the simulation to help motivate her.

While Juliet's ex seems like he may be manipulating her into making him a rich man with her hard work, on the island at least, Juliet becomes something of a manipulator as well. As mentioned earlier,

Juliet tries to cheat for Jack by telling him to kill Ben. Why does she do this? Ben may have told her that if she could cure Jack's issue of having to fix everything, he'd let her go home (surely Ben realizes Juliet will not be able to succeed). Leaving Ben broken—with a tumor—is probably the objective for Jack's treatment since he must always fix everything. Of course, even with Juliet's help, Jack still fixes Ben anyway, proving that he may be a hopeless case.

The Jack fiasco may not be the only time Juliet has tried to cheat her way off the island. It would be a wise move for both the show itself and Juliet if it turns out that she lied about the estimated conception date of Sun's baby. In this episode, Juliet tells Sun that she became pregnant while on the island. The good news about this is that it means her supposedly infertile husband, Jin, is the father. The bad news is that no woman who has become pregnant while on the island has survived childbirth, so Sun will likely die. However, it would make a lot of sense for Juliet to be lying. First, it would help Sun's marriage since, if she hadn't gotten pregnant on the island, it would mean Jin wasn't the father. What the couple doesn't know won't hurt them, right? Second, Ben has told Juliet that he'll let her go home once she is able to prevent the deaths of women who become pregnant on the island. If Sun actually didn't get pregnant on the island, she won't die, and this will make it look as though Juliet's fertility treatment saved the day. Therefore, Juliet can return home. What a stinker.

This twist is actually a pretty good move for the show too. The problem *Lost* begins to have in the third season is that, with all of the interesting character backstory twists already told and the big riddles unable to be revealed until the end of the series, a big gap is left in the middle with nothing to say. I think the original plan was to bring in new characters from the plethora of second-class island survivors and to explore their stories. But after the negative response from Paulo and Nikki, the writers realized they needed to try something else. To keep the storyline intriguing, they created several new twists and mysteries that could be solved before the series ends. I believe they began planting many of these toward the end of season three and will be revealing quite a bit of them in season four—the Juliet lie possibly being one of them. It's an interesting twist and will hopefully be one of many that will enable season four to be considerably more captivating than season three. Here are some other possibilities: Claire and her baby won't be rescued but taken prisoner by the approaching ship; Paulo and Nikki will somehow be resurrected only to die a much more painful death later on; and lastly, Ana Lucia will be dug up and discovered to have been a man.

Still Lost?

Now that I've laid out how all the Losties, Tailies, and miscellaneous misfits fit into the simulation equation, no doubt you still have some questions about some of the other *Lost* mysteries. Like who is Jacob? What's the deal with the four-toed statue? Where are the whispers coming from? What exactly is the monster? And how does *The Lost Experience* play into any of this? For answers to all these and many more questions, stay tuned for the sequel to this book—*The Myth of Lost II: Everything Else You Ever Wanted to Know about Lost,* coming next season to fine bookstores everywhere! Just kidding. I'm not gonna keep you hanging like some *other* forms of media I know. All the big questions about the myth of *Lost* are answered in this chapter. Notice I said the answers to the "myth" of *Lost*. I'm not going to get into the questions about the characters' storylines because that's just up to the whims of the writers. There's no myth on whether Sawyer will end up with Kate or whether Sun ever hooked up with Michael. That's all soap opera stuff. My guess is as good as yours. With the myth solutions, however, I feel that even if you get an explanation from the show, there's still always room for more deliberation on it. So, without further ado, here are some solutions to how the rest of the *Lost* mysteries fit into the simulation theory.

The Others

The role of the Others became clear to me during the first episode of season three when Juliet was revealing to the imprisoned Jack everything she knew about him. She appeared to have an entire case file as though she were his therapist, or was at least playing that role within the simulation. While the true intentions of the Others still remains a mystery, they obviously know a lot about the Losties and seem like they want to help, albeit using rather unconventional methods.

I believe that the Others are a combination of therapists, doctors, researchers, and actors (and possibly even friends and relatives of the patients) that have entered the simulation program with the test subjects in order to help them successfully navigate their way through it. What probably happens is that before entering the simulation, each assistant is assigned to a few "lost" patients. They are paid either by the patients themselves or the government via the rehabilitation program to help them get through their issues and find themselves again.

In order to help the therapists get settled and organized before beginning the session, they probably enter the simulation program a few weeks before the patients and chill in a little community. This way, they can develop their plan on how they will save the next batch that's scheduled to arrive. The Others village that is revealed at the start of season three is this community where I believe the therapists warm up. While they most likely know that a new group will be coming, what they probably don't know is when and how (i.e., plane crash). Immediately after the patients enter the program, the researchers spring into action. Once they do, it makes sense that they play into the faux-reality that the patients believe themselves to be in. For this reason, they dress up as castaways who have been stranded on the island themselves. This is so the patients won't be jolted back to reality upon seeing a bunch of doctors in lab coats in the middle of a tropical island. By initially playing the role of fellow castaways, the therapists ease the patients' transition into the illusionary world.

Now, I assume that not every patient who arrives on the island will get the same treatment. The kids, for example, would likely need to be put into a separate kiddie program just for them—this is why all the children are taken away by the Others early in "the session." The reason Walt isn't abducted originally is because, as previously mentioned, he has been put into the system to get to know his dad. He is later abducted so he can see how much his father cares for him. The answer is "a lot," as his dad risks his life and kills two people in order to save him. Well, the two deaths are probably not a part of the intended father/son bonding process that Michael paid for with his ex-wife's money, but shit happens when you give people freewill (just ask God). All that was probably supposed to happen was that Michael rescue his boy and the two bond quicker than they ever could've in the real world. Once Walt is abducted by the doctors, however, they notice that he has amazing psychic abilities. So they decide to hold on to him a bit longer for some tests. Eventually, Walt is freed, but he isn't the only one to receive extra attention.

About halfway through the simulation session (i.e., the end of season two) the therapists review the progress of the various patients to see who might need some additional treatment. Among the latest batch of Losties, three candidates are picked for this extra help—Jack, Kate, and Sawyer. The reason the Others want them (and put them on Michael's list), is because they aren't really improving. Jack still needs to be in control of everything, Kate is still not following rules, and Sawyer still doesn't play well with others. They need a more intense regimen, hence the "unpleasant two weeks" they have to endure on the Others' island from Ben Linus and the gang. Over the course of the two weeks, the three stubborn Losties are slowly broken—Sawyer with the heart monitor and realizing he has nowhere to run, Kate by learning to follow orders and care for others, and Jack by being in a position where he isn't in control and seeing that some broken things shouldn't be fixed. Seemingly, the additional treatment helps, considering that Sawyer begins to chill out, Kate begins to show real feelings for Sawyer as well as think about someone besides herself, and Jack *almost* chooses to not "fix" Benjamin in order to save his friends—even though those friends include a scoundrel and a chick he likes who's just hooked up with said scoundrel. Obviously, Jack is going to take more work if he is ever going to be cured … assuming he even can be.

During this time, one of the Others—Colleen—is shot and killed by Sun. Her husband, Danny Pickett, is seemingly very upset by this. This is a perfect example of why I think the Others are comprised of actors in addition to therapists and researchers: to help make the simulation as convincing as possible. Danny may simply just be acting upset. In fact, Colleen may not even be his real wife. Another possibility is that some of the Others may not be in on the simulation program deal. Perhaps they have their thoughts manipulated just like the Losties. Whatever the case, the one thing that's for certain is that there is a method to the Others' madness. Their strange behavior is all part of the plan. Everything happens for a reason in the *Lost* world, just like in ours. The difference, however, is that on *Lost* we get to see why seemingly senseless actions or random events are being purposely brought about.

For example, in the third season episode when Jack returns with Juliet to the Losties campsite, Claire suddenly becomes sick. While this seems like a random event, we later learn that Juliet has implanted a device in Claire that infects her with a disease that only Juliet could cure. Once Jack's treatments fail, Juliet springs into action and saves the day, thereby gaining the Losties' trust. This is but one example where *Lost* has shown us that the Others are able to control what seems like natural occurrences. What else might they control? How about the plane crash? Considering the plane splits in half right above their heads, the Others don't seem particularly fazed. Ben has even commented that they have time. Time for what? Obviously, this is planned.

Since the Others have proved to be such effective planners, it seems rather odd that they would build the entire simulation just to cure people's issues. Surely, there has to be a bigger reason for the project. As I've stated earlier, the patient treatments are most likely a way of funding the simulation. Still, I don't believe they are meant to be its main purpose. So what is?

Most *Lost* theories out there assume that the island is an actual, albeit magical, place. According to one theory I've heard, the members of the DHARMA Initiative (the ancestral Others) are trying to change an unfortunate destiny of the world by experimenting with the destinies of unfortunate people. The island is used because its strange properties allow the Others to witness the effects certain key changes have on different timelines or dimensions (similar to the movie *Dark City*). This would explain why the Others need people with issues—to try to clean them up. The problem with this theory, however—besides being exceedingly complicated for your average TV viewer—is that, with the exception of possibly Desmond, none of the characters' flashbacks have gone through any kind of change. And how would this theory explain the monster? Lots of holes, but still interesting nonetheless. If it can be explained clearly, I wouldn't be disappointed at all if this turns out to be related to the final answer. For now, though, I have a different explanation that fits in with the simulation theory.

I think the original purpose of the Lost Simulation was for it to serve as a realistic laboratory to uncover universal secrets. Its main inhabitants—DHARMA—were likely hippie scientists who wanted to conduct unorthodox experiments without the usual constraints of the real world. Within the simulation, they could study the effects thoughts have on virtual reality, how our choices affect others, and how seemingly natural events often help us reach our goals. More innovative studies could have also been conducted, such as the possibility of using the mind to change the aging process, manipulate genetic characteristics, or enable one's consciousness to travel through time and space. Scientists could then take their findings and apply them to the real world, in hopes of making it a better place. Unfortunately for DHARMA, those plans don't work out. Because although they are the main residents of the simulation, they aren't its first residents. Those would be "the Hostiles" as they are termed. I believe the Hostiles are a competing group of doctors, scientists, and investors who probably helped fund the simulation and are, therefore, more interested in the financial rewards—and power—it can provide. So while the DHARMA Initiative came into the simulation seeking harmony and answers, the Hostiles came looking for money and glory. It's easy to see why these two groups were destined to have a falling out.

Initially, the two groups were probably assigned to different parts of the island. DHARMA was given the barracks section, where they could set up their little scientific hippie community. The Hostiles were given (or banished to) the rest of the island to work out their money-hungry schemes. Their first scheme was probably to use the island as a sort of fantasy playground for playboy billionaires (a possible reason for the four-toed statue—part of a Greek gods motif, perhaps?). When that didn't work out, they probably experimented with other possibilities, like offering it up for around-the-world balloon race simulations for people such as the original Henry Gale. Finally, they decided the simulation would be most profitable by treating millionaire mental cases, reforming convicts (on the government's tab), and perhaps even enabling women with problem pregnancies to successfully have babies. They also apparently decided that they'd need the entire island for these plans to work. Hence, DHARMA had to be eliminated.

As we saw from the season three flashback, Ben helps make this happen by snuffing out the DHARMA camp. Of course, they aren't actually killed, just ejected from the program. As the mastermind behind the DHARMA purge, Ben is immediately made king of the Others and enjoys this power immensely. So much so that he decides to expand his kingdom, enabling more and more patients to enter the simulation. Ben's power tripping makes even more sense when you consider that he's most likely a nobody in the outside world. This also explains why he doesn't want anyone to leave.

Much like the Losties, Ben has his own issues. His issue is that he enjoys the little world he's built for himself in the simulation and wants to keep it exactly as it is. To do this, he needs to keep the simulation funding flowing by curing patients. He also needs to continue his leadership position and to prevent anyone from leaving without his okay. Everything Ben does is to accomplish one of these three goals, explaining a lot about his seemingly mysterious behavior. For example, the reason Ben tricks Locke into not pressing the button in the hatch is so that it will blow up and reset the system. The Others later insinuate that this has affected their off-island communications—in other words, they can no longer just beam out of the simulation. Ben has also indirectly led Locke to blow up Mikhail's communications station as well as the submarine, and let's not forget that he let Michael and Walt escape using their only seaworthy boat. Combine all of these events, and the result is that no one can leave without dying. This gives Ben all the more power.

Still, Ben's power to prevent everyone from leaving is useless if he loses his leadership position. As we begin to see during the third season, many of the Others are becoming increasingly unhappy with Ben and are looking for a new leader. Strong, confident, and able to communicate with the island, John Locke seems like a logical choice; and this explains why Ben feels threatened by him. First Ben tries to publicly humiliate Locke by showing the Others his weakness. Unlike

Ben, Locke can't destroy his biggest fear—his dickhead father. Ben feels this humiliation is enough to put Locke in his place. And it probably would have been if Richard Alpert had not come to Locke's aid. Alpert helps Locke cheat by telling him that Sawyer also has a vested interest in killing Locke Senior. So, Locke gets Sawyer to do his dirty work and is redeemed. Why does Alpert cheat for Locke? Probably because he's become all too aware of Ben's hunger for power. He may see in Locke a man who he'd much rather have as leader. Once Locke brings back his father's dead body, Ben really begins to feel threatened. That's why, shortly afterwards, he shoots him and leaves him in the DHARMA mass grave to die. Ben is eliminating the competition. Then again, from Ben's perspective, Locke's act of offing his dad means that he is cured anyway.

Despite Ben letting his ego get the better of him, I believe that he is still the head therapist running the simulation program. For this reason, he is still trying to cure his mental patients despite that they're nearly overrunning the program. This is why during the third season finale, Ben orders fellow Others, Tom and Ryan, not to really kill Sayid, Bernard, and Jin when they are kneeling before them on the beach. The reason is because they aren't ready to leave yet. Ryan reminds Tom that they've been instructed just to shoot into the dirt, but Tom is angry and says that Ben doesn't know what he is talking about. That he's "lost" it. Truth is, Ben has his reasons. Not only would curing his millionaire patients ensure that the money continues to flow, it will also build a good reputation for the simulation program, helping to acquire future rich patients (*Lost II?*). Of course, it also adds to Ben's ever-increasing ego, which he demonstrates whenever he insists that "[he and the Others] are the good guys."

Overall, I do believe that the Others' intentions are good. Whether they are rehabilitating criminals, curing people's issues, or helping women successfully give birth, these all seem like worthy causes. But what of the whole fountain of youth angle? In one of the flashback episodes, we see a very young looking Ben with a Richard Alpert who doesn't look any younger. Even more curiously, Alpert supposedly works for Mittelos Bioscience, and Mittelos is an anagram for "lost time." While there are too many theories about this to list here, I have a couple of favorites. The first is that it's not that Alpert is aging very slowly, but that Ben and possibly some of the Others are aging very quickly. This would explain the age-progressed uterus that Alpert shows Juliet when he comes to recruit her. Another theory is that Alpert and the other Hostiles are the age-delay experiments of DHARMA who escaped captivity. Yet another theory is that the show just does a really bad job of trying to make Alpert look younger. Personally, I feel that there is, in fact, something being done with time experimentation, which I'll address further in Desmond's time traveling section. For now, I'll just leave it as one more convoluted aspect the writers decided to add to an already confusing batch of mysteries.

Speaking of which, one of the reasons I feel the show becomes so convoluted during the third season is because the creators didn't have a timeline for when it would conclude. For this reason, they added in a lot of unnecessary fluff since they didn't know how much time they needed to kill. I think the series suffers a bit from these superfluous mysteries, but with the final episode now scheduled for 2010, I'm hopeful that *Lost* will be able to progress more steadily, and satisfyingly, to its natural (or supernatural) conclusion.

Him

"Him," as the mysterious head Other has come to be known, reminds me a lot of Charlie from *Charlie's Angels*. He's the man calling all the shots, but you never really see who he is. Perhaps an even closer analogy is the wizard in *The Wizard of Oz*. While early on we are led to believe that Ben is the metaphorical man behind the curtain, it is later revealed that this title belongs to someone by the name of Jacob. By the end of *Lost's* third season, in the episode revealingly titled "The Man Behind the Curtain," we finally catch a glimpse of the ghostly Jacob and his impressive telekinetic powers. However, much like the wizard in Oz, Jacob most likely uses tricks and special effects to make it appear as though he is something he's not. So he is probably not the great and powerful invisible ghost he appears to be, but someone much different—an ordinary man who is controlling the illusion of the simulated world.

If the writers are keeping with the myth, the real identity of this man shouldn't be revealed until the end—or, at least, close to the end—of the story. At that point, we will likely learn that "Him" is not one of the characters within the program, but the programmer himself—the guy or gal who created the Lost Simulation. Interestingly, *Lost* gives us a huge hint as to who this might be with their introduction of another character in "The Man Behind the Curtain" episode—Horace Goodspeed.

Horace is the long-haired, good-natured man who tries to save baby Ben's mother when complications arise shortly after she's given birth. Years later, Horace is the one who brings young Ben and his father to Lost Island. This is particularly telling since, in an earlier episode, Mikhail "Patchy" Bakunin mentions that Jacob had brought everyone to the island. This seems to indicate that Horace could very well be him. However, if Horace really is Jacob, why is he called Jacob instead of Horace? Actually, Horace is never referred to by his first name in the episode which he appears. He's known only as Mr. Goodspeed. Perhaps, he prefers to be called by his last or middle name since Horace is kind of old-fashioned, and perhaps his middle name is Jacob—H. Jacob Goodspeed. Could be …

If Goodspeed is Jacob, how could this transformation have occurred? Well, we know that during the DHARMA Purge, Goodspeed is among those killed. Upon dying in the simulation, people are supposed to be ejected back into reality. However, since Horace has such a vested interest in the program, perhaps it doesn't work that way for him. In refusing to leave his project behind, perhaps part of him gets stuck on the island—leaving him in a vegetative or semi-conscious state in the real world and as a transparent image within the simulation. Like a ghost continuing to haunt its old dwelling because it's unable to move onto the next realm, Horace is trapped between two worlds and not fully himself in either. This might explain why he pleads with Locke, saying only, "Help me."

While it is possible for other characters to be Jacob—everyone from a future bearded Jack and wig-wearing Locke, to an older Ben, a broken-nosed Desmond, a messed-up-looking Christian Shephard, or a skinnier Leonard Simms—there is a lot of evidence pointing to Horace. For starters, Ben doesn't respect many people, but upon discovering Horace's body after The Purge, Ben shows his respect by gently closing the dad man's eyes. He does not do this with any of the other bodies. The only other being Ben seems to respect is Jacob, so perhaps they are one and the same. Then there's the fact I just referenced that Horace brought Ben to the island, as Mikhail had said Jacob had done for everyone—another clue? There are also physical similarities. With his long hair and receding hairline, Horace matches the first ghostly glimpse we are given of Jacob's profile. Finally, considering how much attention *Lost* pays to character names, surely the fact that both God and Godspeed appear in Horace's last name—Go(o)dspeed—is no coincidence. Within the simulation, Jacob is revered to be like God. Further evidence of Horace's Godlike status is given by his job title as revealed on his DHARMA jacket—mathematician. In a world created by binary code, who is God? Surely, it is the mathematician.

If Jacob is indeed God within the simulation, then what does that make Benjamin? He's obviously someone of considerable power, controlling the Others, yet he almost seems inhuman in a lot of respects. Funny I should say that. I think it would be a very cool twist if we found out that Mr. Benjamin Linus doesn't really exist—that he isn't based on an actual person in the real world and only exists within the simulation. In other words, Ben could be the human form of the computer running the simulation program, similar to the doctor on *Star Trek Voyager*. On that show, the doctor is a holographic human created by the ship's computer. It could be the same deal here. Ben would be like the computer incarnate—or at least, virtual incarnate—who may or may not know that he isn't real. This would explain a lot about Ben's personality, or lack thereof. It would also explain his high tolerance of pain and inept socializing skills. Also, Ben originally claimed to be the only Other who had lived on the island his entire life. If this is true, it would fit perfectly with this theory since Ben technically would've been born on the island the moment he'd been created. What a great way to throw everybody off. At least, that's what I thought.

Admittedly, season three gives a major blow to this sub-theory when it features a flashback of Ben that portrays him being born in the woods near Portland. While it's possible that this backstory is just a fabricated memory given to Ben to make him think he is real (similar to the fake memories the androids were programmed with in *Blade Runner*), I think this angle is too convoluted for even *Lost* to pursue. Yet, why would Ben lie about being born on the island? To give himself more credence as leader? Perhaps, but what if he isn't lying? What if there is another explanation?

When Richard Alpert first meets Julia, he tells her his facility is located in Portland. It's therefore very possible that the simulation program is located somewhere near there. Since this is where Ben's parents are supposedly hiking during his birth, perhaps they are actually in the program at the time, but either the island hasn't been developed yet, or they're just on a different island. It does seem like they are in the simulation, though, because Ben's mother dies during childbirth, which is one of the issues of the program—pregnant woman die. This would explain why Ben is so obsessed with rectifying this flaw. If this scenario turns out to be true, it means that Ben was, in fact, born within the program, just not on the island. This makes sense since he later tells Locke that he hasn't been born on the island after all. While it seems like a far stretch, I'm gonna stick with my "Ben Isn't Really Real" theory if for no other reason than because I think it would be an interesting twist for his character.

Imagine what a shocking ending for the show it would be to have the *Lost* gang coming out of the simulation and seeing their respective therapists, who turn out to be the Others. At that point, Hurley, or one of the other tricksters, asks where Benjamin Linus is. With a smirk, one of the Others points to the Linus 3000—the computer that has been running the Lost Simulation. They then explain that their nickname for the computer is Big Ben, hence Ben's full name. "Cool," Hurley says. Yes, very cool. In a *Twilight Zone*-ish, creepy kinda way.

The Whispers

The whispers are a group of low-pitched voices that are usually heard in times of danger. Mythologically speaking, they sort of represent our gut instinct—those little voices we sometimes hear inside our heads. Everyone gets those … right? The crash survivors from the tail section of the plane and Danielle Rousseau associate the whispers with the Others, but a direct correlation has never been made. In fact, this false assumption is what leads Ana Lucia to accidentally shoot Shannon—she hears the whispers and panics. Turns out, there aren't any Others after all—just a spoiled blonde chick chasing after the doppelgänger of an abducted little black boy with supernatural abilities. If *Lost* is anything, you have to admit it's original.

So are the whispers from the Others, from the island itself, or from something else entirely? My answer, in a word, is "yes." While the lost patients are in the simulation, I believe they can still hear—on a subconscious level—what's going on in the outside world, including the voices of people talking. You know how they say that comatose victims can often hear people who are speaking around them? It's like that. While the Losties are all lying around on tables with electrodes attached to their heads, there are people working around them in the outside world. Some of these people might be doctors or researchers—other Others. Some of them may be the patients' friends and/or relatives, and some may be the former castaway participants who have "died" and are now out of the system. Whoever these people are, all of them are probably able to watch what's going on in the simulation world and can't help but comment on it—kind of like how some people get at horror movies, warning the young, pretty girl who just lost her virginity not to go into the dark, creepy cellar. If this is what the whispers are, it makes sense that they are heard during tense moments, since it's those times when the audience watching the Lost Simulation is most likely to begin to blurt out advice to the subjects within the simulation. *Hey Shannon—look out! Ana Lucia's got a gun! Oooh—damn! Dying sucks.*

Incidentally, there are actually people out there with enough free time to decode entire episodes of *Lost* using fancy audio software, enabling them to decipher what the whispering voices say. I'm not going to get into the details here. Lostpedia.com has the full whisper transcripts listed if you're interested. Interestingly, however, some of the things the voices are saying when Shannon gets shot are, "here she comes, here she comes," "she likes this guy," and "dying sucks." Oh, and there is also "Hi, sis." I suspect that this one is said by Boone in the real world, once his sister joins him there after dying in the simulation. Just a guess.

Ghosts, Doppelgängers, and Other Strange Visions

Speaking of Boone, many of the Losties see dead people. Locke sees the ghost of Boone; Jack sees an image of his father, Christian; and Mr. Eko sees his dead brother, Yemi. Does the island have amazing energies that allow the dead to appear to the living? Does it make its inhabitants see things, or does the simulation theory have an explanation for all this? I'm gonna go with "C"—simulation theory explanation. And here it is …

According to the simulation theory, when you die on the island, it means you've gotten over your issue(s) and can return to the real world. That would mean that Boone never truly dies. He just leaves the program. So if he's not really dead, it's entirely possible that he's chilling in the outside world, rooting for the patients still remaining inside the simulation, and helping them. The subconscious mind is an amazing thing. Because of this, I believe that if Boone were to talk with the unconscious Locke, Locke would hear his voice (as with the whispers). Since Locke would recognize the voice, the image of Boone would also appear. This explains Locke's visions of the bloody Boone and how they led to his saving Mr. Eko—even if it is only long enough for Mr. Eko to save himself. Ghost number one—solved. But what about ghost number two, Jack's dad, who is dead before the Losties even get to the island. Or is he?

I believe that Jack's dad is alive and well. This belief gets a real boost during the third season finale when Jack keeps referencing his father as though he is still around. Sure, Jack is doped up on drugs and possibly insane, but that's what enables the writers to get away with his rambling statements—viewers can't be sure if he is speaking the truth or not. I'm guessing he is since it fits in nicely with my theory. Remember, according to the simulation theory, none of the castaways were ever really on a plane from Australia, unless they took one from there to DHARMA's simulation facility. Most likely, though, all of their memories were implanted by the program to help them explain how they got to the island. So Jack never really goes to Australia to bring back his father's body. It's all in his mind.

I think Jack's father's death is simply part of Jack's treatment, which his dad may be paying for. I can totally see his father helping him from outside the simulation, and maybe even going in for short periods in order to help him from there. The first time Mr. Shephard does this, he leads Jack to his own coffin—which is, not surprisingly, empty. However, the coffin is near the cave where the Losties set up camp and find drinking water—a key find that changes the course of events. The second time Mr. Shephard's presence is felt is after Jack has flashbacks about his ex-wife. He is the Others' prisoner at this time and tries to communicate with someone using the intercom on the wall. It is at that point that his father's advice squawks through—"Let it go, Jack." He is trying to help his son move forward with his treatment. Ghost two—solved.

On to ghost three—Mr. Eko's brother. This one's a bit trickier. Even the simulation theory states that the reason Mr. Eko is on the island is to come to terms with his brother's death. So his brother really *is* dead right? Right. But then, how could Mr. Eko see him? My answer is that he doesn't. Remember what Yemi says after his brother refuses to confess his sins to him? He says, "You speak to me as if I were your brother." Yemi is a simulation created by the program, just like the drug smuggler's plane where Mr. Eko found his brother's remains. Yemi is programmed in so that Mr. Eko can see him again. Wouldn't it be great if you could say everything you want to say to a loved one who's passed away—especially if he or she died unexpectedly, and, even more especially, if you believed the death was your fault? Even if you knew you weren't really speaking to that person, the act would still help you come to closure. So unlike Boone and Jack's dad, Yemi's ghost is not provided by the real Yemi. He is created from the information Mr. Eko gives the programmers before going into the system. Ghost three—solved. But wait a minute—what about Walt? He is alive and in the program when he appears before Shannon. How does he do that? Good question.

As stated earlier, unbeknownst to everyone including the researchers, Walt has psychic abilities that are enhanced within the program. The program is, after all, connected to the brain. Walt's apparition is different from the other ones since he is not only alive when he makes his appearance (technically making his apparition a doppelgänger), but inside the simulation with everyone else. Remember, Ms. Klugh—the Other—asks Michael if Walt ever appeared in a place where he wasn't supposed to be. This is because they are beginning to discover his power. A power that he's used on the island. So that explains Walt's appearance to Shannon. But what about when he appears to Locke after he's left the island with Michael on the boat?

If Walt is still floating around inside the simulation program somewhere with his dad, then I'd say he's simply using his teleporting superpowers again. If he's managed to get out, he still may be using his abilities to project an image of himself to someone within the system, or he may be watching the progress of everyone he left behind—particularly Locke, with whom he has a connection and would like to see succeed. As with Boone, the sound of Walt's voice may have made an impression on Locke while he was unconscious within the program. Why Walt appears so much older, however, when only a month or so is supposed to have elapsed since he left the island, makes no sense whatsoever. Obviously, the actor playing young Walt hit puberty and began changing. Still, the writers could explain the age difference by stating that time on the island is different than time in the outside world. This may add needless complications though, especially since any time differences would make more sense the other way around—with time going faster within the simulation world, not in the outside one.

Still another possibility to explain Walt's appearance is that, like Yemi, Walt may have been a projection of the simulation/monster. Then again, this still doesn't clarify why he looks older. Chalk it up to the constraints of reality, I guess. What *is* clear is that Walt represents the wishes of the island (the simulation) when he appears to Locke. In an attempt to stop Naomi's approaching ship from arriving, Walt's doppelgänger somehow saves Locke from the pit so he can stab Naomi in the back as she's contacting it. The island is either protecting itself from the threat of the ship (as Ben states), or it knows the remaining subjects are not yet ready to leave the simulation. Either way, season four will tell if this action is successful, but I have a feeling it is too little, too late.

Well, that explains the ghosts and doppelgängers of Lost Isle, but what of the other strange visions, like Hurley's imaginary friend Dave? He doesn't even exist. Ah, that's a horse of a different color. Speaking of which, what about Kate's horse? That's a horse of the same color as Dave. Both Kate's horse and Dave, I believe, exist only in the minds of Hurley and Kate, respectively. What Dave tells Hurley in the Lost world is true, however—none of it is real. Dave tells Hurley that if he kills himself, he'll wake up in the real world. According to the simulation theory, this is absolutely true. As stated earlier, in most

107

mythology, ghosts and visions usually speak the truth, and such is the case with Dave.

With Kate's horse, I believe it's almost like her guardian angel. We first see the horse in Kate's flashback, when she is being chased by the marshal. The horse is in the middle of the road, which causes the marshal to swerve and hit a tree, enabling Kate to escape. Does it really exist? Is this the first time the horse has been in Kate's life? I'll let the writers answer those questions. As of this writing, they have yet to do so, but I think that the horse must be pretty significant in Kate's life. Perhaps it represents a stuffed animal she had as a child and confided in when trying to hide from her alcoholic father. Or maybe it is a real horse she used to ride at a stable somewhere. Regardless, the horse provides an escape for Kate from her troubled youth. This would explain why she sees it immediately after Sawyer has channeled her father whom she'd killed. Speaking of which, what is going on there? Is her father really alive? Is he possessing the weakened body of the dying Sawyer? Or is one of the researchers in the outside world just messing with her? I'm gonna go with none of the above. I think Kate's guilty conscience is just seeping into her subconscious. Just a guess though. And one that probably doesn't matter, because I think it's one of the minor mysteries that the *Lost* writers will leave unsolved.

Black Rock

"Black Rock" is first mentioned by Danielle Rousseau to Sayid when she is holding him prisoner. Technically, the very first time it is mentioned is in Rousseau's French-spoken distress signal, but you have to understand French to catch that since it's never translated by Shannon. As we come to discover, Black Rock isn't a rock at all, but a ship—an old slave ship that somehow managed to get beached very inland on Lost Island. The discovery of the ship, combined with the stories of other wrecks (Danielle's and Desmond's, as well as the crashed planes and other aerial transportation vehicles such as the hot air balloon), leads viewers to believe that the island is some kind of Bermuda Triangle—trapping hapless traveling victims in its magnetic clutches. What really amazes me about the show is how well the writers' leads (most likely false) about the island's magnetic abilities and the simulation theory fit so well together. Yes, it makes sense that all of those boats and ships and airplanes crashed on the island due to some strange electromagnetic force. But what makes even more sense is that all those vehicles haven't been there all that long—that they all served as a means to believably transport the test subjects and therapy patients into the simulation without their suspecting anything odd about how they'd arrived on the island. Even if that's so, however, why an old slave ship? Who would want to arrive that way? There's only one person I can think of, and he most likely would have been the first candidate to test the effectiveness of the therapy treatment of the simulation program. That person is Alvo Hanso. Alvo Hanso of the Hanso Foundation—the foundation that backed the DHARMA Initiative.

According to *The Lost Experience*—the alternate reality game based on *Lost* (that I don't necessarily subscribe to as being factually tied in with the series but will accept its information in this case)—the Black Rock was owned and operated by Magnus Hanso, grandfather (or possibly great-grandfather) of Alvo. Both Magnus and his ship disappeared in 1881 with Magnus presumably at its helm.[10] Now, since the ship is on the island, it seems to be a pretty strong argument against the simulation theory. If the ship really disappeared in 1881, then it disappeared in the real world. If it's on the island, it would seem that the island is real—unless Alvo created the ship, and possibly the entire voyage, in hopes of recreating what might've happened to his grandfather. The virtual island that the ship crashed on within the simulation program is where Alvo decided to set up camp for future DHARMA research since he felt that this island would have magical properties—even within the simulation. Sure, it's kind of convoluted. But can you imagine *any* scenario explaining all the details of the many *Lost* mysteries *not* being convoluted at this point?

Another possible reason Alvo might have wanted to recreate the Black Rock would be to help him come to terms with the fact that he owes his family fortune to the slave trade. Just as Mr. Eko brings back his dead brother to come to terms with his life, perhaps Alvo does the same with his dead grandfather. And after being cured of his guilt, he decides to help others do the same by financially backing the initiative. This explanation is no crazier than a nineteenth-century slave ship disappearing at sea only to end up landlocked in the middle of a magical island no one could find from the outside world. Actually, it's a lot less crazy than that, which is why I'm sticking with it. In fact, even if the show comes to explain that the ship really landed on the island, I'm still gonna say that the mythic aspect of the story would say otherwise. It's all an illusion. Just like life.

The Statue

One of the most memorable lines of *Lost* has Sayid saying, "I don't know what is more disquieting—the fact that the rest of the statue is missing, or that it has four toes." A four-toed statue. It doesn't seem to make sense, no matter which *Lost* theory you subscribe to—but certainly not for the simulation world. If the island is all a simulation, why would someone have created a giant statue, only to later destroy it?

First of all, who's to say that the entire statue ever existed at all? Perhaps it was designed to make people think it was part of something bigger—a scarecrow of sorts to scare test subjects away from that part of the island or to add to the seemingly inexplicable mystery of the island itself. That's possible, but within the realm of the simulation, why create just the foot of a statue when it's just as easy to build the entire thing? One reason could be that the original test subjects weren't supposed to see the mysterious statue too early in the experiment, that it was meant to be discovered later once they had advanced through other tests. While this is also possible, I think that at one time the entire statue did actually exist, and that its purpose predates any of the experiments that took place on the island. In fact, I think the statue is as old as the island itself.

Before we get into why the statue might've been created, let's break down the mythology of it for a moment. The idea of a giant statue rising out of the ocean to guard a land mass extends as far back as the Colossus of Rhodes. One of the Seven Wonders of the Ancient World, the Colossus was a gigantic statue of the Greek god Helios that stood at the entrance to the harbor of the Greek island of Rhodes. It's been said to have inspired the Statue of Liberty and Emma Lazarus' famous poem, "The New Colossus," which is carved into Lady Liberty's base.

So the mythology of this statue seems pretty well ingrained in our collective unconscious—but why four toes? Is this to suggest that it was created by another species of man? An alien race? An ancient tribe who worshipped cartoon characters that are infamous for having eight fingers and eight toes? While all feasible explanations (well, except for the cartoon character one), none of them really fit with the simulation theory. However, there is another possibility. It's well known in archeology circles that many ancient people signified the divine and supernatural nature of their gods by creating statues of them with an abnormal number of appendages. It was a way to set their gods apart from mere mortal men. So mythologically speaking—which is logically the route to explore since this is the realm in which *Lost* operates—the statue would seem to be of some kind of god. Great, but why? Could the Lost Simulation originally have been designed as a mythological Greek island or interactive computer game, complete with gods and goddesses? Maybe, but I think there's a less expected and more interesting possibility.

Let's think realistically for a moment about the type of people who designed the simulation program. They would be brilliant, well read, creative, devout fans of videogames, and most likely possessing a very sophomoric sense of humor. In a word—nerds. Now, considering that they are spending all of their time creating this simulation world, isn't it logical to assume they'd have a little fun with it now and again? Perhaps creating little hidden gems, or "Easter eggs" as they are more commonly known? And in some cases, might they also create a few obvious fun things just for shits and giggles? Things like, oh, I don't know, a giant statue of themselves as a god to be worshipped by whoever came to the island? Or, perhaps Alvo Hanso had commissioned such a statue of himself as a joke, or not as a joke, depending on his ego. Either way, the statue would have most likely been destroyed so as not to confuse early arrivals on the island. But, perhaps the programmers decided just to leave the foot as a memento. Or, maybe they figured no one would ever venture that far, so it would be one of those hidden Easter eggs.

In order for this explanation to be correct, the creators of the show would have really needed to have done a lot of in-depth thinking about some seemingly minor details that don't have much to do with the main storyline. Does this seem at all likely? Hell yeah! Have you been watching the same show I've been watching? Realistically though, I freely admit that this theory is unlikely to end up being the one that explains the existence of the statue, and the writers may very well come up with a fascinating explanation that is mythologically sound. Still,

I think this explanation is likely to be more fun than any they might come up with. And after taking this show so seriously, I think we could all use a little fun.

As far as other explanations, I've heard that there are a lot of literary references made about similar statue appendages that exist out there. One of the better ones is from a book by Thomas Love Peacock called *Headlong Hall* which says: "Here you see is the pedestal of a statue, with only half a leg and four toes remaining: there were many here once." Very similar, no? The thing is, even if the *Lost* writers do borrow from these references, they most likely do so to help with the story details, as opposed to the overall mythology. So the questions of whether Jack is based on the protagonist from a Stephen King novel or if Sawyer's situation comes from a theme of *Watership Down* are unlikely to help solve *Lost*'s big questions. Yes, the writers provide hints by occasionally featuring the covers of various books that inspired certain story elements, but these hints are unlikely to give away much. They are just for super zealous fans who like exploring every possible aspect of the series. Perhaps, someone like you. And to a much lesser extent, me.

The Eye

As mentioned previously, I realize that many of the explanations I'm describing here may end up being different from what the writers ultimately come up with. Still, that doesn't make the overall simulation theory wrong, just the details, of which there could be many versions that might still fit within the overarching theme. One theory I especially liked concerning a mystery of the show, indeed, ended up being incorrect, as far as I can tell. That theory attempted to explain the rationale for showing the close-up of a character's eye before his or her flashback or at the start of certain scenes in which the character is prominently featured.

The eye has always seemed like a fairly obvious signature element of the show, but to my surprise, a lot of people I've spoken to about it had no idea what I was talking about. If you are one of these people, the eye usually appears just before a character's flashback. For a few seconds, we see an extreme close-up of that character's eye that allows little else to be seen. The pilot episode actually begins with just such a close-up of Jack's eye dilating. When I first started noticing the eyes, I figured that they served as a stylistic and intriguing way of delving into a character's past, without any real meaning behind it. I soon began to look deeper into the meaning behind the eye, however, when I noticed that not every flashback began with the eye, and sometimes the eye was shown without a flashback—as with Jack at the start of the first episode. So I began to wonder why it was sometimes being shown and sometimes not.

After paying attention to when the eye did and did not show up, I came to the conclusion that it indicated a fabricated memory of the character created by the simulation. If the simulation theory is correct, then some of the memories the characters have would have to be fake—created by the simulation—while others would be real. This concept is very similar to themes explored in movies like *Blade Runner*, *Eternal Sunshine of the Spotless Mind*, and *Total Recall*. In this case, the computer would have implanted memories to make sense out of how the Oceanic Flight 815 survivors got to the plane and, for that matter, got to Australia to begin with—assuming the simulation facility is not located there.

Why show an eye? In the real world, the test subjects of the Lost Simulation are likely sitting or lying down with electrodes attached to their heads that are connected to the main computer that's running the program. A way to convey that a particular flashback is fabricated by the system could be to show the character from *outside* the simulation right before the flashback is shown. This way, we are reminded where the character actually is and conclude that it's the computer creating the memory. Doing this would make clear which memories are real and which have been artificially induced. Problem is, if the creators were to show the characters strapped in chairs, it would give away the entire *Lost* mystery. So instead, they just show the character's eye, which could very well be open at times while they are undergoing the simulation treatment. This method also allows for a cool revelation once the truth is exposed. Imagine seeing a close-up shot of Jack's eye. Then, the camera slowly pulls back, allowing us to see where he really is—in a *Matrix*-like apparatus with wires coming out of his head. Woohoo! Yet another mystery explained by the simulation theory! But then, during the start of the third season, something happens to kill this explanation.

It happens at the start of Locke's flashback, shortly after the hatch explodes. As with other flashbacks, we get to see a close up of Locke's eye, only something is different this time. The shot isn't as close as usual, enabling viewers to see more of his head—a head that is cut up and bleeding from the explosion. While it's possible that Locke's head somehow got cut up in the real world outside the simulation and that this serves to create his delusion of the hatch exploding within the program, I decided to abandon the theory. I just didn't think the writers would needlessly throw us off a path that has barely been explained. Still, it is possible that the eye close-ups do serve to differentiate which flashbacks are real and which aren't, but I no longer feel that they are showing the character's face from outside the simulation. Too bad, because I really liked that idea of zooming out from a close-up of Jack's eye to reveal where he and all the other Losties had actually been all along. It would allow for *Lost* to come full circle. Dagnabbit, why am I not writing for this show? Their explanation better be jaw-dropping good!

Mikhail "Patchy" Bakunin

Known for the trademark patch he wears over his right eye, Mikhail Bakunin is a member of the Others with a rather Michael Myers/Jason-like ability to be seemingly unkillable, that is, until he is apparently blown up by his own grenade at the end of season three. Mikhail (or "Patchy" as fans like to call him) makes his first, rather creepy, appearance on a black-and-white TV monitor within the Pearl station early in that same season. Archetypically, Mikhail's patch is most symbolic of a pirate—and what do pirates do? They live outside the rules of society so that they might carry out their desired lifestyle of pillaging and plundering booty. In other words, they're seafaring anarchists. Interesting, considering that Patchy's namesake is Mikhail Alexandrovich Bakunin, a Russian revolutionary known as one of the founders of modern anarchism.

A nineteenth-century anarchist philosopher, the real Mikhail Bakunin rejected government, authority, God, and the concept of a privileged class. While this obviously seems to be a good fit with your typical pirate, what insight can it provide about Patchy? For starters, working in relative isolation at the Flame communications station seems to suggest that he separated himself from island politics and even the governing Others. A self-described loner, Mikhail likens his job to that of a lighthouse keeper and enjoys working by himself while keeping tabs on the outside world with his array of TV monitors. These monitors provide him views of various spots on the island, as well as access to the world beyond. It is this access that gives us the true insight into Mikhail's pirate motif. As someone who has direct contact with the outside world, he is quite simply above the laws of Lost Island. In fact, this just may explain his incredible ability to continually reincarnate himself after being left for dead several times on the island.

After running through the Others' electrified fence, Mikhail experiences convulsions and blood dripping from his mouth before collapsing to the ground, seemingly dead. Is it all an act? The trembling could've easily been faked, and biting his tongue could've gotten the dripping blood effect. That was my first thought; however, I now believe Mikhail does actually "die" and then return. He may even pull the same trick after taking a harpoon to the chest courtesy of Desmond, only to appear again soon after—this time with a grenade that he uses to blow a hole in the underwater Looking Glass station. While that explosion seems to take Mikhail's life yet again, and the *Lost* creators assure us that this time he's really dead, who knows? The real question, though, is how he manages all these death-defying feats.

Once again, the simulation theory has the answer. Thanks to Mikhail's unlimited access to the real world, it is entirely possible that he's been able to download himself back into the program whenever his character—or avatar—is ejected. However, with the Swan station destroyed, the Flame station and submarine having been blown up by Locke, and the Looking Glass station flooded, Mikhail may finally be out of methods to return to the simulation. This could be why Damon Lindelof confirms that Mikhail is officially dead, but I'm sure they can find a way to bring him back if necessary. Perhaps with the as-of-yet-undiscovered Earth, Wind, and Fire station?

Until meeting his third and presumably final demise, Mikhail actually plays a very important role for the Others. As the liaison to the outside world—even within the context of the show—he is Ben's go-to man for securing the information needed to get inside the Losties' heads. How he manages to come by this information, however, is another Mikhail mystery that has yet to be explained. The day the Losties arrive on the island, Ben takes Juliet to see Mikhail, who seems to be viewing reports of the missing Oceanic airliner and gathering data about everyone on board. While this is what we are led to believe, a few things just don't add up about it. To begin with, researching every member on that flight would be a rather overwhelming, if not impossible, task for one person to accomplish in a short amount of time, especially considering all the detailed information the Others eventually wind up with. Even if it were possible, how could Mikhail know that Sawyer had hunted down and killed a man in the middle of nowhere or that Jack's ex-wife was now truly happy? Surely this personal information isn't gathered from Google. Yet these and many more private facts are reported by Juliet, who presumably hears them from Mikhail.

Here's what I think was really going on: while it appears that Mikhail is watching news footage of the missing Oceanic plane, I believe he is actually downloading fabricated reports—or even creating them himself—to add to the believability of the whole plane crash story. He also could just be trying to fool Juliet, who may not be in the know about the simulation. As far as his amazing ability to gather tons of information about the passengers in mere minutes, I don't believe he is searching for this data at all. Why would he have to when it has already been gathered from the patients in the research facility where the patients are all hooked up to the simulation? Surely they would've needed to answer some personal questions before entering the program. And if they didn't provide the information themselves, then their friends, relatives, or whoever brought them to the facility could have. (This is very similar to the research collecting scene in *Eternal Sunshine of the Spotless Mind*, where Jim Carrey's character has to answer a bunch of questions before having his mind erased.) All Mikhail really has to do, then, is to get this information from his contact in the outside world who has already collected it. Whether this is a somewhat senile Jacob, a real or computerized Ben, or some other member of DHARMA, I can't say. What I am sure of is that Mikhail isn't able to uncover Locke's dysfunctional relationship with his father, Jack's compulsion to fix things, or Mr. Eko's guilt about inadvertently causing his brother's death from their MySpace pages.

The Looking Glass Station

The Looking Glass is the underwater DHARMA station that Ben had claimed was flooded, but wasn't. That is, until Mikhail blows out one of its portholes with a grenade. Water immediately floods in and drowns poor Charlie only moments after he's deactivated the jamming signal inside. So where's the mystery? For me, the question isn't why Ben lied about the Looking Glass being flooded—obviously he just didn't want anyone going down there—but what it was originally used for. Some have theorized that its purpose was to guide the submarine to the island, yet this seems a bit too obvious for *Lost*, and would it really be necessary to build a gigantic underwater station just to send out a homing beacon? If any station on the island was acting as a sonar lighthouse, it was probably the Flame—after all, Mikhail did say that he felt like a lighthouse keeper. So if the Looking Glass station's purpose wasn't to guide the sub, then what was it? I believe the writers actually give us a clue.

When Charlie is trying to break the code to turn off the jamming signal, he comes to learn that the solution is a musical note sequence to a song. He also learns that the code was originally programmed by a musician. Considering how effective DHARMA was at assigning job titles, why would they want musicians working in an underwater station? This might be a minor point, but I believe that DHARMA had them working on certain frequency experiments, and this was why the station is underwater. If this is the case, obviously these experiments would not be dealing with the money-making psychological treatments of mental patients, but with the bigger, world-saving tests DHARMA was working on within the simulation. Being underwater would enable them to either separate frequencies from those of the island or simply study their visual effects as they moved through liquid. The clue the writers give that seems to be the tip off is the name of the song Charlie has to play to break the code—"Good Vibrations."

Purgatory?

Soon after *Lost* premiered, many viewers began to suspect that the castaways had died in the plane crash and were currently residing in some sort of purgatory, awaiting judgment as to their fate. While this seems like a very plausible theory, the show's creators adamantly denied it, leaving fans wondering what other answer there could possibly be. For the first couple of seasons, the show steers clear of any purgatory references. Then, toward the end of season three, all that changes when a couple scenarios hint that the castaways might be in hell or purgatory after all. Have the show creators been lying, or is this just yet another attempt to throw fans off the trail? Let's examine these scenarios and see if we can come to any conclusions.

It is Locke's father, Anthony Cooper, who reveals the first bombshell when he is held captive on the island. "Don't you know where you are?" he asks a dumbfounded Sawyer. He then says, "Wherever we are, it's too hot to be heaven." Since the writers choose a despicable con man to imply that the Losties are all in hell, this is a pretty sure sign that they really aren't. But then, how does Cooper get there? He claims that he was in a car accident, and next thing he knew, he was on the island. I'd say that he only thinks he's been in a car accident because that's what the simulation causes him to believe—assuming it's even really him. Like Eko's brother, Mr. Cooper could be a trick of the monster created to help Locke and Sawyer get over their issues. Either explanation makes more sense than the Losties being in hell, because if that's the case, how has Penny made contact with them? That's just one of the hundreds of problems with the hell theory, while so far there are really only two arguments for it. The appearance of Naomi on the island leads to the second one and is just as easily debunked.

Toward the end of season three, Naomi Dorrit parachutes onto Lost Island after her helicopter begins malfunctioning. She claims to work for a company that was hired by Penelope Widmore to track down Desmond, whom she has a picture of. Upon learning from Hurley that she has wound up on an island with the survivors of Oceanic Flight 815, she seems confused and tells him that Flight 815 had been recovered and that there were no survivors. Say what? Even creepier, while talking to Charlie, Naomi realizes he is the rock star whose body was supposedly found in the wreckage. Assuming Naomi is telling the truth, how could all the survivors of Flight 815 have been found dead, and yet be living on the island, if they aren't in some kind of afterlife? Actually, there are three science-fiction precedents that provide some interesting possibilities.

The first is the *Twilight Zone*-ish or *Donnie Darko*-like alternate dimension explanation. For this explanation, a plane is caught in some kind of Möbius loop or dimensional rift that causes it to enter multiple timelines. In one timeline, the plane crashes, but not in the timeline where we've been following the passengers and crew. They are stuck between worlds. Sometimes they return, and sometimes they don't. Since *Lost* does touch on time travel themes and has given hints about "lost time," this could very well wind up the explanation to what seems like contradictory storylines. But I doubt it, since it is not simple enough to be satisfying.

Another explanation involves the ol' switcheroo. As seen in the movie *Millennium*, passengers who are about to die in a plane crash are kidnapped by future beings (or aliens) and replaced with realistic doubles (or real corpses). In *Millennium*, the reason is because mankind is impotent in the future, so they have to go back in time to kidnap people who are going to die anyway, so as not to change their timeline. Mix this concept with USA Networks' *The* 4400, and you get a theory where the DHARMA Initiative is a group of scientists from the future who try to save the world of their time by creating an artificial island that exists in the past but acts as a gateway to their dimension. The sentient island gathers together certain individuals whose future actions will bring about the destruction of the world, and changes these people so that the world is saved. A cool theory, but I don't think *Lost* is going there since it's even more complex than the first explanation.

The third possibility is that the passengers were never actually on the doomed flight at all, but that the crash did, in fact, occur. This fits pretty well with the simulation theory since it could mean that the fake plane crash the Losties experience has been based on one that has actually happened in the real world. The benefit of doing this is that it would provide the simulation programmers news reports and footage from a real crash, adding to the believability of the experience. Then they'd just have to make the Losties think that they'd been on the plane by implanting fabricated memories, and they'd have the beginnings of a convincing simulation. A bit complicated, but it works. Still, all three of these theories assume that Naomi is telling the truth about the recovered wreckage of Flight 815, but I don't think she is.

Until we receive more information about the supposed rescue ship and its crew in season four, it's difficult to predict exactly who they might really be, but I have a couple very plausible thoughts. My first is that they are programmers and scientists from the real world who will attempt to take back the simulation program, which has clearly gotten out of control. This explains why they're looking for Desmond, since he's in there against his will. The members of the crew may even be law enforcement officials or DHARMA. Whoever they are, they probably are not going to take too kindly to what's left of the Others.

I alluded to my second theory about the "rescue" ship earlier in the Desmond section, claiming that it was sent by Penny's father, Charles Widmore. If this is the case, the crewmembers will most likely want to prevent Desmond from ever leaving, so he could never marry precious Penny. This would not only explain why Naomi has the picture of Desmond and Penny, but why she would lie about the Losties all being dead. If you're living on a tropical island and find out you're dead, would you risk leaving, not knowing where in hell you might wind up? Probably not. The devil you know is better than the devil you don't.

Another reason I think Naomi is lying is because her discussion with Charlie has too many holes. She claims to have been from the same hometown as Charlie yet doesn't seem to have ever even heard of his band. She only knows that there was a "dead rock star" found among the casualties of the doomed Oceanic flight and that his former band had released a greatest hits album in his memory, which had sold very well. Even if she isn't up on her pop culture, the Losties were only supposed to have been gone a few months by then. Are we to believe that Charlie's body was discovered, they had his funeral, his bandmates decided to put together a greatest hits album, and that it sold very well, all within that time frame? Okay, *maybe* if it was only released on iTunes, but otherwise, I'm not buying it.

Whatever the explanation, I'm definitely not buying that the *Lost* gang is dead. How would this theory explain the numbers? The contact with Penelope? The flash forwards with Kate and Jack and whatever other flash forwards we get in season four? Most important, *Lost* isn't going to uncover its big mystery until the very end. It's the mystery that keeps viewers watching. Perhaps originally, the Losties were supposed to be dead, but once fans figured it out so quickly, J.J. and Lindelof had to change the whole solution. Let's all hope this didn't happen.

Everyone's Connected

Very often, one of the castaways or one of their friends or relatives appears in the flashback of another castaway. For example, Hurley somehow appears on TV in Korea winning the lottery in Jin's flashback, Kate's mom—a waitress—serves Sawyer in a restaurant, Kate's adoptive dad is in Iraq with Sayid, and Jack chooses to operate on his future ex-wife, Sarah, instead of Shannon's father, both of whom have been in the same car accident. Jack's decision costs Shannon her father, and with it, her family's money. Why all the connections? Mythically speaking, this is the writer's way of expressing their belief that all of us are connected somehow—interlocking gears in the clock of life. In fact, *Lost* creator J. J. Abrams even went on to create another show, *Six Degrees*, in which this theme is even more prevalent.

The "everyone's connected" theme is more than just a cool concept for movies and TV shows, though. It taps into a spiritual truth that we are all really connected in our own lives. The idea is that outside of the illusion of this material world we live in, we are all really one—one energy, one life-force, one light, one God—whatever you want to call it. This is what the myth of *Lost* is ultimately attempting to convey, whether you agree with it or not. Chances are however, if you don't agree that we're all connected, you probably don't like, or even watch, the show. If you'd never really thought about this possibility before but do watch the show, you're probably more open to it now, thanks to *Lost* subliminally working its magic on you. This is the power of mythology.

While the connections between the various characters on *Lost* may just be a statement of the writers with no real relevance to the plot, according to the simulation theory, it can actually be explained. Perhaps the lives of everyone on the island seem to be connected because they are all physically connected in the outside world—patched together with wires and plugged into the system. In other words, the simulation program could be grabbing memories from one person's mind and splicing them with another's, or each test subject in the simulation could be subliminally pulling the memories together themselves. So

Hurley isn't *really* on TV in Korea—Jin's memory of the TV being on is just spliced with Hurley's memory of being on TV. And Shannon's dad doesn't really get passed up by Jack for emergency treatment—that image is created by combining both their memories of a middle-aged man dying from a car accident. To borrow a theme out of *Star Trek*, all the castaways are like the Borg. They're all connected, and that includes their minds and memories.

From this perspective, then, there are probably very few real connections that actually happen between the Losties. It's all just been mixing of memories, with the archetype of one character being substituted for another. For example, Nadia—Sayid's lost love—represents the damsel in distress because this is who she is in his mind. Sayid had helped Nadia escape from the Iraqi Republican Guard after he was ordered to have her executed. Since Sayid's memories are connected with everyone else's, Nadia plays the same role in their minds as well. So in Charlie's flashback, the image of Nadia is substituted for a woman he rescued from a mugger—the same damsel in distress motif. She even calls him a hero. For the record, Nadia means "delicate" in Arabic.[11] This is indicative of the role she will play in everyone's memories.

Most of the connections on *Lost* happen within character flashbacks. Yet, since there really is no difference between a memory and the virtual reality of the simulation, these fabricated connections can happen on the island as well. So Locke's father, Anthony Cooper, probably isn't the same person as the con man who killed Sawyer's parents. This is just one of those connections the simulation brings about since the archetype of a con man in both Locke and Sawyer's minds registers as one person. Since they're living in their thoughts, so to speak, and sharing the same "dream," Locke's idea of his father is able to fit with Sawyer's idea of the man who killed his parents. Within their illusionary world, Anthony Cooper is able to fulfill both roles. Either that, or—as previously theorized—he is a trick of the monster and just tells Sawyer what he needs to hear.

Obviously, this is all just a theory, and there's really no evidence on the show that the Losties' memories are being merged together. Or is there? In one of Desmond's flashbacks, Charlie is seen playing guitar on the street for money, and Desmond approaches him just as it begins to rain. Interestingly, Charlie has a very similar flashback of himself playing guitar on the street for money when, suddenly, it begins to rain. Only this time, there is no Desmond. And the location is different. So perhaps the street musician Desmond encounters isn't actually Charlie after all. What happened is that Charlie's memory of himself playing guitar on the street merges with Desmond's memory of some random street musician playing in similar conditions. Desmond probably can't remember what that musician looked like, so the simulation fills in the blank with an image from Charlie's memory. Since they're connected, their memories connect.

In most cases, the numerous character connections that have happened on the show can be explained in this way. However, there are a few instances where I would say that the intermingling of castaway memories *do,* in fact, occur—but just not as we see them. For example, I do think that Libby actually meets Desmond—I just don't think she gives him a boat. What she gives him is information on the simulation program. But as with a dream, Desmond's subconscious translates that thought into something that can be understood in his present reality. Either that, or the computer changes that memory for him. Does Desmond really meet Jack at the stadium, then? Perhaps. But more likely, that is a flashback memory provided by the *Lost* program. Whatever the details, it certainly makes more sense than all of these chance encounters happening purely by coincidence. There are no coincidences. Everything happens for a reason in our world, and *Lost* usually tries to show that. I hope that the writers won't brush off all these connections without some sort of logical explanation. The simulation theory works for me. If not, the writers have a lot of explaining to do, and the explanation cannot be that *everyone is connected in real life, so that's what we did on the show.* The show is a metaphor that's meant to make concepts like this understandable to the audience. This is one of the reasons why the simulation theory fits so well.

If you do not subscribe to the simulation theory and instead believe that everything that's happening on the island is actually real, then not only do you have to explain why they are all there and what the hell's going on, but you also have to explain how it is that their lives are all connected. I mean, how is it that Kate's mom just happens to serve Sawyer, who just happens to bump into Jack's dad, who just happens to meet Ana Lucia, and on and on. Explaining all that would be quite a challenge. It is actually very possible, however, to explain how everyone's connected using any variant of the previously mentioned "life as illusion" theories—such as the version where the entire Earth is an illusionary program, and the Lost Island is its central mainframe. With this version, everyone is connected because the Lost computer makes it that way. The purpose would be so that they would all eventually end up on its shores, possibly to repair it, help run it, or whatever the computer's motives would be.

In short, explaining how everyone's connected by using a theory that has all the main characters in some kind of an illusion is easy. Once you believe that everything on the island is really happening, though, it becomes a lot trickier. I'm not saying it can't be done, just that it might take a lot of backstory. And with so many unanswered questions on the show, who needs more confusing explanations as to why things are the way they are? The Losties' memories are all connected because their minds are all physically connected. It's that simple. And when it comes to any *Lost* explanation, simple is good. Very good.

Desmond's Time Traveling and the Skeletons

While most mythological stories are content exploring one or two hidden truths of our world, *Lost* takes on a whole slew of them. The ideas of "life's challenges making us stronger," "the universe revealing clues about our destinies," and "everyone being connected" have all been central themes of the show. Another major theme, not really discussed yet in any detail, concerns the illusion of time. The illusion of time is a belief that forms the basis of many myths. It is talked about in numerous spiritually themed works and in those of quantum physics as well. According to the illusion of time theme, everything that has happened, will happen, or could happen is all happening at this very moment. While this may seem a bit complicated, basically, any story that features any kind of time travel is illustrating this theme.

Lost gives us many little hints about time related issues. First, we see one of the Others reading Stephen Hawking's book *A Brief History of Time,* which discusses space/time wormholes among other things. Then there's the name of Richard Alpert's company, Mittelos, which is an anagram for "lost time." Another hint is given during the brainwashing scene with Alex's boyfriend, Karl. One of the messages he is listening to says, "Only fools are enslaved by time and space" when played backwards.[12] All of these little clues are fun, yet there's definitely a much bigger message concerning time that's woven into the plot of the show. Having been the focus of many episodes, Desmond's time traveling exploits are the most obvious.

As previously mentioned, I believe that when Desmond turned the fail-safe key of the Swan station (causing that weird noise and purple haze), he rebooted the Lost Simulation program. Now I'm going to add an additional possible twist. Perhaps more than just resetting the program, he resets time within it as well. The result of this is that Desmond witnesses all the possible scenarios of the program as it is being reloaded. This explains how he could see into the future. It's almost as if he's played the Lost game already and hit the reset button to play again. Now he already knows what the game is. In fact, this explanation for Desmond's prophetic abilities is pretty much confirmed during the "Flashes before Your Eyes" episode.

In this episode, Desmond (wearing an extra-long, multicolored scarf reminiscent of fellow time traveler, Dr. Who) seems to relive certain key moments of his life while still having the knowledge that he's already lived them before. This enables him to predict everything that is going to happen. It works exactly the same way on the island. The reason Desmond is able to see the future is because he's already lived it. He isn't *predicting* events, he is *remembering* them. Within the simulation, being able to do this seems possible since it's all just a program, but how does Desmond replay events from his actual life? The answer is he doesn't. He just replays the memories of his life—memories as they would appear while he is still connected to the simulation.

This explains why the beeping of the microwave in his old apartment sounds exactly like the countdown timer of the computer in the Swan station, why the song that comes on the jukebox in his hometown bar is the same Mama Cass song he used to play while on the island, and why the numbers (and the Oceanic flight number) make an appearance when a delivery man brings in a package for room 815. As just mentioned, it also explains how he just happens to bump into Charlie playing guitar on the street. Different elements from Desmond's memories that are somewhat similar (beeping microwave and beeping countdown timer) are merging together, making them seem connected. It's the same explanation as to why everyone on the island seems connected through the people that they know—different people from the Losties' memories who have similar characteristics merge together, making it seem as though someone from one person's life is showing up in another person's life. The simulation is substituting similar archetypes and symbols for one another. Sounds crazy, yet this also explains the strange symbolism we get in our dreams that really represents other things—things our mind is unable or unwilling to process. Once again, *Lost* is trying to explain a truth of our world.

So, if Desmond's flashback is all in his mind, this begs the question, who is the old white-haired lady who won't sell him an engagement ring? In the episode, her name is Ms. Hawking—yet another nod to the physics of time and to Stephen Hawking. She comes across as a sort of omniscient being, telling Desmond that his fate is set in stone and that he is not meant to be with Penny. So who is this Negative Nancy? Is she Desmond's conscience? Some random dream character? Jack's grandmother? I believe her image is likely someone from Desmond's subconscious (she is seen in a photograph with the monk who Desmond worked with at the monastery), yet her words are coming from the computer simulation. If Penny's dad did force Desmond into the simulation program, he likely also set up some safeguards to assure he wouldn't leave. Convincing Desmond that pushing the button is the most important thing he'll ever do is one way to do that.

Mythologically speaking, Ms. Hawking is God. She's omniscient, after all—knowing both Desmond's fate and that of the man with the red shoes who had a scaffolding collapse on him. While I don't believe Ms. Hawking is really supposed to be God, I do believe she is speaking the truth from the perspective of the simulation. Within that realm, the destinies of the various characters are pretty much set in stone. They have one path they can take to win—that's it. On this path are multiple challenges they must conquer to move to the next level. And they will repeatedly be given these challenges until they pass them. So Charlie is repeatedly tested with the drugs, Sawyer with his temper, and you, with the issues that keep coming up in your life.

Speaking of repeating tests, one that has been given to all of the Losties is actually given to them again shortly after Desmond resets the system, presumably because they failed it the first time. This is the teamwork test. Early on in episode one, Boone jumps into the ocean to save a young blonde woman who is drowning, but winds up needing to be saved himself by Jack. Because of this, the woman died. After resetting the system, Desmond jumps into the ocean to save Claire. He later claims that, had he not done so, Charlie would have jumped in instead and drowned in his attempt. Perhaps the simulation is giving the Losties another chance to work together, or perhaps the simulation is simply repeating a challenge since Desmond reset the game. Either way, it is a demonstration of history repeating itself and déjà vu—yet more real-world truths portrayed on *Lost*.

Getting back to the broader "illusion of time" theme, while not as obvious as Desmond's time traveling abilities, I believe the skeletons found in the cave during season one also illustrate it. Dubbed "Adam and Eve" by Locke, the skeletons just may be the key to the entire *Lost* mystery. In interviews, Damon Lindelof and Carton Cuse claim that the skeletons will provide proof that they knew what the end of the show was going to be right from the start.[13] While this statement may be meant to throw us off, I think it's legitimate. This being the case, who, then, are the skeletons?

Well, in order to prove any kind of twist ending (which is pretty much par for the course for *Lost*), the skeletons are most likely two characters that are still alive when the skeletons are discovered. The most likely choices are Kate and Sawyer or Kate and Jack. The reason any of these characters would make sense, according to the simulation theory, is that none of them may be curable. For this reason, they will probably never be killed on the island, and, therefore, will never be able to leave the simulation through traditional means. Instead, they will be forced to spend their whole virtual lives there (maybe about one year in real time) until they "die" of old age or starvation. Only then will they leave the simulation ... uncured.

This may explain the flash-forward sequence from the end of season three (discussed in more detail in that section) showing Jack back in the real world in really bad shape. Since Kate is there too, perhaps they are the last two to escape the system. Or, maybe they find a way to escape without solving their issues and then try to return, becoming skeletons in the process. Regardless of the details, which I'll leave to the writers, there's definitely a chance that the skeletons are Jack and Kate. Still, the fact that Locke refers to the skeletons as Adam and Eve seems to give more weight to Sawyer and Kate. Both have committed sins that they must pay for in the outside world, and both have partaken in tasting each other's forbidden fruit.

Certainly, Jack and Kate or Sawyer and Kate seem to be the obvious choices for the skeletons, but if there's one thing *Lost* isn't, it's obvious. Deciphering the myth of the show does not allow me to predict the specific details of its future events, just how those events might be explained. In the case of the skeletons (which I believe is the name of either a Hardy Boys or Encyclopedia Brown mystery), it is very possible to explain how they came to be using the simulation theory, but there are many ways to do so. My favorite takes into consideration that Desmond really does reset the system, and therefore time. After the reset, whatever originally brought about those skeletons may now not have even happened yet. So, getting back to the scenario just mentioned, if Jack and Kate manage to return to the simulation after having escaped—since Desmond reset time—it may now be earlier than when they first crashed there. If they successfully "die" during this return visit, then they will become the skeletons that their past selves will eventually discover once time catches up to the plane crash.

It all sounds pretty confusing, but it's actually just like a video game. Suppose your buddy Desmond is playing a game and kills off some characters that must die in order to clear a level, then you join in and see the corpses he left behind (this is a very graphic video game). If you later reset the game, those characters are still alive but must eventually be killed. It's a similar idea here, except *Lost* is playing off the concept that time is an illusion, so it's almost as though everything is actually happening simultaneously (which many followers of quantum physics believe to be the case in our world.)

While the simulation theory can explain time warps, should this concept become more prevalent on *Lost*, the alternate dimension theory mentioned during the purgatory section is probably the more suitable theory to use. According to this theory, the magnetic energy of the island may have caused Flight 815 to somehow be thrust into a different timeline. If it sent the plane into the future, and Desmond's actions managed to set time back to the past, then Jack and Kate could return to the island *before* the plane crash had occurred. Then they would die and become the skeletons. The plane would crash, and their corpses would be discovered by their past selves. While interesting, I feel that this solution could get too confusing for the average TV viewer, especially since it would also have to be used to explain all the other mysteries on the island. Plus, I feel like this "time rift" direction has already been done many times before—most recently with *Donnie Darko*, which even involved an airplane and jelly-like creatures not unlike the smoke monster. Stephen King's *The Langoliers* also explored the idea of airline passengers going through a time rift filled with mysterious happenings and creatures. The only real benefit of this theory is that if Jack and Kate somehow manage to return to the island *much* earlier, then we might get to see how all the DHARMA stuff on the island came about. Of course, they'd probably have to stay in the cave the entire time or they would end up in Ben's pit with the rest of DHARMA. This might explain why they die there.

Using either the simulation theory or the alternate dimension theory, Jack (or Sawyer) and Kate seem to be the most likely candidates for the skeletons, but they aren't the only ones. Since the skeletons are likely a couple, there are many more to chose from. Perhaps Jack returns to the island alone where he finds Juliet, and together they live there for the rest of their days. Or maybe Penny eventually tracks down Desmond, and they both stay on the island—away from Penny's meddlesome father. Rose and Bernard can also end up as the skeletons, particularly by plugging into the simulation theory. The two of them seem to have made their peace with the island and may plan on living there until the end. With Rose's illness, leaving the island will mean certain death, and since Bernard loves her, he'll do anything to make his time with her last as long as possible. So, they'll likely "die" there … together. This result might have even been decided upon before Rose and Bernard ever entered the system, so perhaps the skeletons were already programmed in, explaining why they are there from the start. They also may have disappeared since Desmond reset the system.

My final vote for the skeletons is Nikki and Paulo. These misfits were so unpopular that the writers decided to kill them off shortly after they were introduced. Yet the show's creators had originally promised that Nikki and Paulo were supposed to play a very important role in the *Lost* myth. Since they're now both dead, what role can they possibly play? Unless … *they* are the skeletons. Perhaps, but if not, what exactly was their purpose on the show? And are they truly dead? If you don't care about either, simply skip the next section.

Paulo & Nikki

I believe that the original plan for *Lost* was to slowly introduce the minor castaway characters, like Dr. Arzt, as the regulars were killed off—which they would be once their stories had been fully told. Doing this would enable the show to run indefinitely and stay fresh without having to portray all the survivors of the plane crash from the get go. This explains why the writers chose to even have any survivors that were outside of the main group at all. Brought into focus during the third season, Paulo and Nikki quickly proved that this plan was not going to work.

When Paulo and Nikki were first introduced, the *Lost* creators claimed that they were going to play a major part in the solution to the show. Since then, they have admitted that the duo was a blunder.[14] Still, I'm not so sure. Well, I'm sure that the writers' attempts to make them fit in with the rest of the gang and try to get us to care about them didn't work out. What I'm not so sure about is that their appearance on the show will amount to nothing. Paralyzed by spider bites and mistakenly thought to be dead by the Losties, Nikki and Paulo are buried alive on the beach. Perhaps they will never be heard from again, but I believe this is a grave mistake (pun intention not specified). For starters, neither of them solve their issues, and this completely contradicts the message (and precedent) of the show. Perhaps this could open the door for a spin-off series, *Lost II—Resolving Issues*, in which those characters who don't get cured the first time around revisit the simulation with the audience—this time, aware of what's going on. Since this is unlikely to happen, their purpose for being on the show does seem to be in question. Unless Nikki and Paulo aren't really dead after all.

In typical *Lost* fashion, the show has provided several hints that Nikki and Paulo may eventually be resurrected. The most obvious occurs during Nikki's flashback scene when we learn that she has guest-starred in a fictitious TV show called *Exposé* before arriving on the island. Shortly after her character is killed off on that show, Nikki is walking with the producer, who tells her that they could always find a way to bring her character back (wink, wink). Then there is Locke catching Paulo in the act of burying his stolen diamonds in the sand. Locke tells him that nothing on the island stays buried for very long … as in their dead bodies, perhaps? There are many ancient myths where a dead body buried in the ground is reborn as a changed being. Maybe this is to be the fate of Nikki and Paulo. Locke has also mentioned that the winter tides dig up whatever is buried on the shores, and in the same episode, Nikki says it had just been Thanksgiving, so winter is obviously approaching. Real hints or red herrings? Time will tell, but unfortunately, it's probably the latter.

Even though they aren't particularly interesting characters, I hope Nikki and Paulo aren't dead since that would contradict the patterns—and mythology—that *Lost* has created. In fact, with the sole exception of their premature deaths, everything else about Nikki and Paulo fit those patterns to a T. For example, just as all the other castaways are either exceedingly wealthy, directly connected to riches, or criminals, so are Nikki and Paulo. They fit best into the criminal category, yet since they may have gotten away with their crimes, they fit into the wealthy category too. Either way explains how they could've ended up in the simulation—they bought their way in or were forced in for behavior modification. Another similarity between these two and the other castaways is that they have some pretty deep issues. In their case, they both only care about themselves, to the point that they would kill someone they know intimately, just for their money. And just like the other castaways, they are tested on the island to see if they can overcome their issues.

An example of this is when Paulo discovers the Pearl station while trying to find a hiding place for his stolen diamonds. During the five minutes he is down there, Juliet and Ben just happen to walk in, discuss their dastardly plans regarding Jack, Kate, and Sawyer, and walk out, without ever noticing Paulo, who's overheard everything. Oh, and they also "accidentally" leave one of their walkie-talkies behind. Considering how aware the Others are of their surroundings, is it more likely that this slip-up is all a coincidence or that it is a test for Paulo? A test which he fails. If he cared about anyone other than himself, he would have told the other castaways about what he'd overheard, about the station, or at the very least, about the walkie-talkie. But no, he keeps it all to himself. Probably so he can keep the location of his stolen diamonds a secret.

My feeling is that if Paulo and Nikki are indeed dead, and stay dead, then the writers have caved to network pressure and public opinion, corrupting the spirit of the show. Without a soul, *Lost* will be, well, lost, and continue to drift aimlessly through seasons four, five, and six, becoming ever more convoluted and contrived. On the other hand, should these two numbskulls be dug up by say, the ghost of Walt, his dog, or the ocean tides—and be resuscitated—then I'd have to say that the show is still on track with its mythology. Having heard that the actors who play Nikki and Paulo did not have their contracts renewed for the fourth season, however, I'm not feeling too optimistic.

Deadly Pregnancies

If there aren't enough mysteries on *Lost*, during the third season, a few storylines bring yet another one into focus—that no woman who becomes pregnant while on the island lives through childbirth. Apparently, this is why Juliet, a fertility doctor, is brought to the island. Since she's been able to successfully help get her cancer-stricken sister pregnant, Ben thinks she might have some luck with their problem cases as well. To our knowledge, only Danielle and Claire successfully live through the deliveries of their babies on the island. Both of them, however, had become pregnant off the island. Sun is the next woman to attempt to give birth, and she supposedly became pregnant on the island. As previously stated though, I believe Juliet is lying and that Sun had become pregnant before arriving. Her lie means that Sun will likely live after giving birth, Jin will believe the baby is his, and Juliet will be able to go home. A pretty neat outcome.

So, why can't mothers live though childbirth if they become pregnant on the island? Seems like it will be a bit of a challenge to explain, doesn't it? Is the island acting the role of the stereotypical slasher flick psycho killer—offing those women who dare to engage in intercourse while in its presence? But then why not kill every woman who has sex on the island as opposed to just those who became pregnant? No, that's not it. Is it that the island can't support any new life, so when a new one comes, another must die? That doesn't work either, because then why would those who conceived off the island be allowed to live? All right, then maybe it has something to do with the magnetic energy of the island or its strange time-warping properties. Eh, too technical. Well, how would the simulation theory handle this mystery? Ah-ha! I thought you'd never ask!

There are at least two explanations as to why this is happening within the simulation. The first is that all the women who have tried to give birth have had issues in the outside world and are brought into the program to try their luck there. It's not the island that's preventing them from successfully having babies, it's a problem they already have. Ben and the gang are just looking for yet another source of income to keep the program running. *Come to the Lost Simulation! Proven to rehabilitate criminals, cure mental cases, and even enable those couples who haven't been able to have children to do so! Rates start at just one hundred thousand dollars!* The idea is that without the issues of the real world, perhaps these woman will be able to give birth. At least, that's Ben's idea. Having supposedly lost his own mother, perhaps he's become obsessed with being able to help would-be mothers within the simulation and feels that with just a bit more experimentation, it could happen.

Admittedly, this explanation is a bit sloppy, mainly because it doesn't have anything to do with whether or not the women become pregnant on the island. While I'm sure I could easily work around this somehow, I'd rather introduce another explanation that I believe makes much more sense within the parameters of the simulation. According to this second theory, women cannot conceive and bear children within the simulation because … it's a *simulation*!! If a woman goes into it pregnant, fine, she can then have a baby in the outside world, which can be patched up with some electrodes à la *The Matrix* and brought into the system. However, if she only has sex within the simulation, she won't be able to have a real baby, only a virtual one. This likely breaks the simulation spell and causes the mother to wake up back in the real world. A mother knows her baby and simply won't accept a simulated substitute. Since Ben wants to keep everyone within the simulation—and under his power—it's in his best interest to try to prevent anyone from dying without his consent. So, he brings in Juliet, hoping that she can find a way to keep the mothers alive and in the system. Since the Lost Simulation is patterned after the real world, it makes sense that Ben would seek the help of a fertility doctor. To date, however, Juliet has not had much luck. And unless she steps outside the simulation and artificially impregnates the women, I don't think she ever will. That's why she needs to lie about where Sun became pregnant. Otherwise, she'll never be able to leave. Considering that Ben doesn't ever seem to ever get any action himself, this may actually be all part of his plan.

What's with All the Daddy Issues?

It's no secret that many of the characters on *Lost* have major daddy issues. These include Jack, Kate, Locke, Hurley, Ben, Alex, Claire, and Walt, to name a few. Similarly, much like a typical Disney cartoon, many of the characters have lost or even killed their fathers. These include Jack, Kate, Locke, Ben, Claire, Shannon, and Sawyer. Why do all the good cowboys have daddy issues? Has J. J. Abrams been repressing some unacceptable feelings toward his own father and used his stories as vehicles to express them? I guess we'll have to wait for the *True Hollywood Stories* episode for that juicy tidbit. In the meantime, I think we can explain the reason for all the daddy issues by chalking it up to psychological cliché.

According to the simulation theory, all the Losties are on the island to get over their issues. And hating daddy is definitely one of the most prevalent ones, at least in TV Land ... and psychology 101. So, the writers just go with the usual example. The repressed hatred of one's father (by males) is known as the Oedipus Complex, borrowing its name from the famous Greek tragedy. In classic psychology, repressed hatred must be purged from the subconscious in order to alleviate its symptoms. One does this by bringing it to the conscious mind, coming to terms with it there, and finally disposing of it. Sound familiar?

The reason Locke's father and so many of the daddies have been eliminated is because the Lost patients are purging them from their minds—"killing" them so to speak. Exorcising their demons. This is how the patients will eventually be cured, assuming they don't go leaving the program too early, as Jack does. Face your fears and hatred and cleanse yourself of them—this is what Dr. Ben is trying to get all the Losties to do, which explains why he *really is* one of the good guys (whether he's the computer program incarnate or not).

In the real world, I don't think most of these dads are really dead— they are just being eliminated from the Losties' subconscious minds. This includes not just those killed on the island, like the dads of Locke and Ben, but those who supposedly died earlier, like Jack's father. Even before the season three finale, I felt that Jack's father was really alive and still do, even though this is up for debate. There's also the possibility that Kate's stepfather isn't really dead either, that she just needed to kill him off in her mind. If this is the case, she won't be a criminal after all, just a mental patient who needs to put her daddy issues behind her.

Season Three Flash-Forward Finale

"What the hell?" That's what a lot of fans were thinking at the end of the *Lost* third season finale. In that episode, we find out that Jack is in a deep depression, addicted to drugs (which he steals from the hospital), heavily drinking (when he can't score the drugs), and contemplating suicide. To make matters worse, this all occurs *after* he leaves the island! How can this be? No one wants to see the guy they were rooting for—the hero—not only lose his battle but become a drunken asshole. It goes against the myth, and it goes against every fiber in our bodies to have to watch this occur! Despite my doubts about whether the writers truly get the entire myth they are creating, I'm sure that they at least understand the consequences of demeaning their hero—a hero audiences have been following for years. Therefore, despite being a flash-forward, the *Lost* story cannot possibly end with the fall of Jack. The proper mythological order is: rise, fall, resurrection. The flash-forward reveals the fall, and it does so brilliantly. Truth is, this episode restored a significant amount of my faith in the path the writers are taking, because the way it is concocted is sheer genius. My renewed faith is why I know that the scene from Jack's future is definitely *not* going to be the end of Jack's story.

With that major issue out of the way, the next logical question is how this episode could possibly fit into the simulation theory. Jack is seen trying to find the island on maps. He speaks about receiving golden pass airline tickets that he and Kate (and possibly the other Losties) are given because of what they have been through. And he uses the tickets to try to locate the island from high above the Pacific. Surely then, the island *must* be a real place. Not necessarily. I still believe that it is not real and that the crash never happened. In fact, I believe it even more now.

Since the flash-forward is just one piece of what lies ahead for Jack and Kate, we were left not knowing exactly how they got off the island. Are all the Losties rescued by the ship that was approaching? That is the implication since the off-island flash-forward is featured in the very episode where the rescue is supposedly about to occur. Ah, but is that just what the writers want you to believe? I say yes. I don't think that they will be rescued so quickly—at least, not all the Losties. What I do think is that Jack and Kate will abandon their fellow castaways and leave before either of them are really ready to exit the simulation. This is why Jack, at least, is so messed up in the future. Everyone else who allows the simulation to run its proper course will be cured. If Jack and Kate join Michael in leaving before they are meant to, their issues will not be fully resolved. So in at least one possible scenario, the simulation theory fits in pretty well with the third season flash-forward finale— but then, how do you explain those points just mentioned that seem to contradict the theory?

For starters, we see that Jack has become obsessed with returning to the island. He has marked-up maps and atlases all throughout his apartment and claims to have taken lots of overseas flights hoping that one would crash and he would wind up there again. So, does the island really exist? I still say no. Obviously, Jack is mentally unstable. The island has become his holy grail, and like the holy grail, it will not be found within the realm of reality. This makes perfect sense because if the island is a real place and the rescue ship really arrives, why wouldn't Jack be able to find the island again? If rescuers could find it once, surely they should be able to find it again. Having only been given that glimpse of Jack's future (as of this writing, this is the last episode that aired), I cannot state with any certainty whether Jack finds out the truth about the simulation or not. But I can make sense out of his behavior either way.

Let's assume that Jack *does* find out that the island is just a simulation. Since his time there, Jack has slowly begun to lose his grip on reality (living a life of illusion for long periods can do that to you). Drunk, depressed and abusing drugs, he's gone into complete denial. He's just snapped, refusing to accept the truth—that there's no going back to the simulation. Most likely, he and Kate leave before they overcome their issues. It's also possible that the entire simulation program is destroyed or corrupted soon after, so that no one can ever return. Just as Jack had refused to accept that his life with his ex-wife was over and tried to get her back, he also tries to do the same thing with the island. As he sinks deeper into depression and psychosis, Jack becomes convinced that he can find the simulated island in the real world, even though he knows deep down that it doesn't exist. This is why Kate gives him such a sorrowful look after he rambles on about going back there—she realizes he is chasing after an illusion. Incidentally, during this scene at the end of the episode, I find it interesting that Jack keeps tapping the side of his forehead as he describes his goal of returning to the island— as though he knows deep down it only exists in his mind.

This theory totally fits Jack's personality profile. He *would* absolutely refuse to believe that the island isn't real. He is a man of science, remember? Finding out he's been living in a fantastical world would be too much for him to take. The other possibility of course, is that Jack somehow leaves the simulation without ever learning the truth. There's a million ways this could happen. One scenario is that while in the simulation, he escapes on the ship, which sinks, and he wakes up in a hospital bed, none the wiser. Perhaps the government doesn't want him to know about the simulation project and created similar disaster scenarios with all its inhabitants in order to get them out. The powers that be may even mess with the subjects' minds to make them forget all about their island experiences; however, this is pretty unlikely. Personally, I think it's more interesting if Jack does find out about the simulation and refuses to accept the truth, but the theory still works either way. That is, if I can explain the golden pass tickets that were given to Jack and possibly all the Losties. How does he get ahold of those if he was never in a crash?

Just as the *Lost* writers have become experts with messing with the minds of the characters on the show, they've become equally adept at messing with our minds. When viewers hear Jack mention "the golden pass they'd given us," most of us assume that the airline has given it out to the Losties as an apology for their traumatic experience. According to Jack, the pass enables him to fly anywhere for free. While this "airline gift" explanation makes perfect sense, it is not the only possibility that explains where the pass came from. Note that Jack does not say that the tickets were given to them by the airline. He simply said, "they," which could be anyone—particularly DHARMA.

If Jack and Kate do have to leave the simulation before they are cured, it would make sense that DHARMA would give them something to make up for their failed experience and any inconvenience it may have caused them. One inconvenience would likely be a newly instilled fear of flying, which could've been a side effect of the simulation. In fact, after the conclusion of the experiment, perhaps it is discovered that all the Losties are inadvertently conditioned to fear flying. This scenario would actually be very similar to what happens in *A Clockwork Orange*, which *Lost* has paid homage to several times. In the film, a convicted criminal is conditioned to feel sick around violence, but is also unintentionally conditioned to get sick when hearing classical music, since it has been playing during his treatment. If the Losties are the first group to experience the plane crash scenario, it's likely that many of them experience this unfortunate side effect and are therefore awarded the pass to nullify the effects. Repeatedly flying would positively reinforce the relative safety of flying, helping to eventually alleviate the newly developed phobia.

Obviously, these scenarios are all merely conjecture. The point is, however, that just because a character says something, doesn't mean you should necessarily interpret its meaning at face value. Especially on this show, where the writers are deliberately trying to mislead us. Yet since *Lost* teaches us to look for clues, perhaps it is possible to use its own wisdom against it. A big clue that goes mostly unnoticed in the season three finale is the physical appearance of Jack and Kate. Jack is seen sporting a full beard, and "Freckles" appears completely pale and freckle-less. While these features are probably chosen simply to make the characters appear older, interestingly, they'd also fit the profile of how someone might look after being strapped down indoors for several months or longer. Since the wonders of modern makeup offer many options to make characters appear older, why lose Freckles' freckles? And why make her look so pale if she's supposedly been on an island for so long? For that matter, why isn't she in prison? Do the authorities feel bad that she's been stuck on a tropical island with a bunch of hot guys for a year or so? Is she still on the run from the law? Simulation theory would suggest that either she didn't really kill her father, as previously discussed, or the correctional program she experienced fulfilled her debt to society. It might even suggest that the flash-forward is part of the simulation, but I'm not gonna go there.

A more obvious clue from this episode is Jack referencing his father as though he were still alive. Due to Jack's agitated and drunken state, we assume that he is either being sarcastic or just delusional. I believe he is neither, and his father *is* still alive. Not only that, I also believe that Papa Shephard is responsible for getting Jack into the simulation to begin with. He probably saw that his son was desperately in need of help and signed him up for correctional treatment—treatment which obviously did not succeed. Now in the real world, Jack is trying to come to grips with the fact that his months spent on the island were an illusion. An illusion no one in his life knows about. Even if it turns out that the wreckage of Flight 815 is found, as Naomi claims, that still doesn't mean that the crash actually occurred. What it *does* suggest is that a real-world alibi was needed to explain the disappearance of all the simulation test subjects and that a pretty rich and powerful person had no intention of them ever really returning. Perhaps then, Ben isn't such a good guy after all.

J-something 'ntham?

Upon realizing that Jack's flashback is actually a flash-forward, it's interesting to then go back and rewatch the episode, looking for little clues that might uncover the bigger mysteries. For example, since Jack is flying on Oceanic airlines, it's safe to say that the airline does not shut down as *The Lost Experience* has stated. That's a pretty big clue since it not only tells us that the airline is still around, despite a supposed devastating crash, but that not everything on the interactive *Lost* game is aligned with the story from the show. In other words, it's not canon.

In addition to the clues like this one, the third season finale also introduces several new mysteries. I've already discussed my thoughts on Jack's father being alive. There is also the mystery of who Kate has to return home to—Sawyer, her baby, one of her ex lovers—who cares?

It's all soap opera stuff. The mystery I am most interested in is one which just might be able to connect the flash-forward pieces to the rest of the *Lost* puzzle: who's in the coffin?

During Jack's flash-forward, we see him reading a newspaper obituary that gets him so upset, it drives him to the brink of suicide. He later goes to visit the funeral parlor where the deceased is being held and sees the funeral director, who tells him he's the only one who's come to the viewing. He then asks Jack if he is a friend or family member of the deceased. Jack tells him, "neither." After the director leaves, Jack puts his hand on the casket looking deeply upset, takes a pill, and walks away. Later, when Jack meets up with Kate, he takes out the newspaper clipping and hands it to her. As she's reading it he says he'd hoped to see her at the funeral. Kate, looking bewildered, hands him back the clipping and asks why she would go to the funeral? So, who do Jack and Kate mutually know that would have no friends, yet whose death would drive Jack to nearly kill himself?

The most popular guesses are Michael, Ben, Sawyer, Locke, and possibly Jacob. While a long shot, there's also the possibility that it's Charles Widmore, since he doesn't seem like a particularly nice guy. One other possibility I'd like to throw out there is Kate's father—the one she supposedly killed but was possibly just a mind trick of the simulation. While I'm throwing this theory out there, it's not my top pick since Kate's dad doesn't seem to be someone whose death would upset Jack. In fact, none of those candidates would. Unless Jack isn't actually upset about losing the person physically, but the information he was carrying—information on how to get back to the island. Whoever is in there, I'm betting that this is the reason Jack is really upset, and this makes a pretty strong case for Ben.

If Ben is in the coffin in the real world, obviously that blows my "Ben Is Actually the Computer" theory, but let's look at the evidence anyway. As far as we know, Ben has no friends, including Jack, which would explain why no one shows up for the viewing. Yet Jack would likely be upset over Ben's death since he'd be his last ticket for getting back to the "island"—whether he realizes it is a simulation or not. With Ben dead, all hope would be lost for Jack ever returning. That's why he'd want to kill himself after Ben's suicide—and yes, it may have been a suicide. According to some fans who've studied the newspaper clipping closely, the obituary seems to describe a man who was found hanging from a beam in his apartment. Considering that Ben spent so much of his life as an important person within the simulation, if it were destroyed and he had to live his life in the real world where he is a nobody, I think that would be grounds for him to commit suicide. Especially since he has absolutely no friends. This makes a pretty good case for Ben being in the casket, except the clipped obituary supposedly mentions something else that poses a problem—that the deceased had left behind a teenaged son. If that's correct, it doesn't seem to fit Ben, who has no son as far as we know. Yet it would fit Michael.

Not only does Michael have a son who'd be a teenager by 2006 (roughly when the flash-forward took place), he's also from New York, which is clearly stated in the obituary clipping. Slightly less clear, but readable, is the name of the deceased. While the name does not appear to be Michael's, this can easily be explained. If Michael has never found out that his island experience was all a simulation, he likely thinks that he really killed Ana Lucia and Libby (until he bumps into either of them in one of his flash-forwards, which would be cool). Believing that he is a murderer who abandoned all the Losties, Michael might very well take on an alias to protect himself. Riddled with guilt and having left the simulation before he was truly ready, it is also possible that he would have been suicidal. Assuming Jack also left before he was ready could explain why he is heading toward a similar fate, particularly if—like Michael—he lets everyone down, too. So, Ben and Michael seem to be the two most likely candidates for the coffin. Perhaps more telling than who's actually in the coffin, however, is that person's supposed name according to the obituary.

Looking closely at a high-resolution image of the obituary clipping, we see the name of the deceased looks like J-something 'ntham. This is interesting because like many of the key *Lost* characters, there is an Enlightment-era philosopher who shares a similar-sounding name. Jeremy Bentham was a philosopher and social reformer whose work led to the development of liberalism. One of Bentham's more important contributions was his design for a prison known as the Panopticon.[15] The concept behind the prison is that it would enable someone to observe the inmates without them being able to tell if they were being observed or not—just like cameras in department stores or pretty much everywhere these days. This feeling of constantly being watched would convey a sense of an "invisible omniscience"[16] and, according to Bentham, enable "a new mode of obtaining power of mind over mind."[17]

Observing prisoners without their knowing they are being observed? As they would be in, say, a simulation perhaps, where they would be psychologically analyzed from observers in the outside world? Very interesting. So if Jeremy Bentham—or a similar sounding name that alludes to him—is indeed the name of the person in the coffin, this would seem to be a big nod to the validity of the simulation theory. It would also seem to suggest that either Ben or Jacob is in the coffin since they likely had a hand in creating the methods by which the simulation would work.

After fans began obsessing over the information in the newspaper clippings, the *Lost* producers announced that it should be disregarded since they were going to rewrite it. So, is the information inaccurate? Was the name of the deceased never meant to be seen? Is the fact that the name sounds like that of a famous philosopher just a coincidence? Perhaps, but what does *Lost* teach us about coincidences? There are none. Even if the writers didn't plan the similarity, the universe could've played a part in giving us a clue. For example, there is another interesting real-life candidate who could've been the inspiration for the name in the obituary. That person is the famous conceptual artist, John Latham, whose art demonstrates the relationship between the past and the present that he calls "Flat Time."[18] Since *Lost* often concerns itself with similar concepts, it's possible that Latham is the namesake of the coffin-dweller whose death has Jack so upset. If this is the case, as with Jeremy Bentham, it implies that the deceased is someone who had a major role in the development of the simulation program. Whichever character does turn out to be in the coffin, though, is really irrelevant to the mythology of *Lost*. The symbolism of this person's death is what's really important.

The message we are getting is that, whoever died, all the good that the island simulation is supposed to accomplish has gone with him. It appears then that not just the castaways, but all of humanity, may be lost. As I said, this flash-forward is hopefully *not* where the story will end. Because if the shamanic superpowers of the creators have been in tune with the energies of our futures, this ending seems to suggest that things are not looking too good. Then again, perhaps *Lost* is serving more as a warning than as an outright sign of things to come. And perhaps, much like the Ghost of Christmas Future, it gives us this bleak ending as a glimpse so that we might change our ways before it's too late. We are subliminally being instructed to stop the hate, the violence, the fighting, the greed, the prejudice, the selfishness, the pollution, the abuse, and the focus on the false idols of the material world. This may be the rationale for the dark glimpse we get into the future of the hero's journey. Or, maybe it is all just a desperate attempt for the writers to gain back some of the show's eroding audience. I'll let you come to your own conclusions on that one.

The Monster

If it weren't for the monster, chances are you and a few million other viewers would have stopped watching *Lost* after the pilot episode. Without the monster, the show, at the outset, is basically *Gilligan's Island* meets *Survivor*. Boooor-ing. The writers knew it was going to take awhile before they could get viewers involved in the complicated story, so they had to create something in the early episodes to keep everyone intrigued. That is most likely why the monster was created. As previously stated, the monster was originally meant to kill Jack, and not the pilot (as in the airline pilot, not the TV pilot, though it was not meant to kill that pilot either). But nobody liked that ending. I give credit to the writers for trying to be unpredictable and going against cliché, but there's a reason those clichés exist—we like them. They are based on myth, and that's what we like about stories—that they speak to us.

If you kill off a character right after viewers have begun to identify with him, where does that leave the viewers? Talk about lost. So it was a wise move to substitute the airplane pilot for Jack as the monster's first and bloodiest victim. Well, *technically*, the pilot is not the monster's first victim. Should you be fortunate enough to own *Lost Season 1* on DVD, pop it in and go to the scene in the first episode where the passenger standing in front of the jet engine gets sucked in and sliced to smithereens. If you watch in slow motion, you'll see a wisp of black smoke slither onto the right-side of the frame and push him in. Apparently, that guy didn't need to be in the simulation. The show creators have denied creating the monster for that scene. But if they didn't do it, who did? Perhaps, it was the *real* monster! Or, a result of bad special effects as they claim.

Danielle Rousseau has described the monster as a security system, and I agree with that assessment. Every once in awhile, the writers try to confuse us by telling us the plain truth. This is also the case with Hurley's imaginary friend Dave, who tells Hurley that the island is all an illusion and that he simply has to kill himself to get out. By mixing in the truth with fiction, the writers leave the audience not knowing what is real and what isn't. I believe that the monster's purpose is to serve as a sort of checks and balances system to make sure no one goes nuts and starts killing everyone, like Rousseau probably did. In fact, the monster may have been created as a direct result of her actions. Or, perhaps one of the test subjects lost it from within the system.

Think about it—some of these folks are paying good money to be in the simulation world. There would be too much of a risk to allow one person to blow it for everybody—hence, the rationale to develop something within the program to take anyone out who begins to display unruly behavior. This security measure could also provide a way out for test subjects once they've completed their mission, (e.g., Mr. Eko). The first time the monster comes face to face with Eko, it does a scan on his memories to see if he has overcome his issues. This is why we see his life flash before his eyes, so to speak. Obviously, the monster decides he has more work to do. (The memory scan may also explain how the monster is later able to transform into the likeness of Eko's brother.) The second time they meet, however, it is time for Eko to go—he's come to terms with his brother's death and no longer feels responsible. So the monster provides for his removal, forcefully ejecting him from the program.

On the blast door map within the Swan hatch that Kelvin Inman (Desmond's former hatch partner) had painted, it mentions "Cerberus" several times. To discover what this could mean, we once again turn to our friend mythology. In Greek and Roman myths, Cerberus is the three-headed watchdog that guards the door to and from Hades' underworld. Translated into *Lost* mythology, Cerberus is the monster or security system that guards the passage of people between the virtual world and the real one. The map refers to the Cerberus having had a "possible catastrophic malfunction" back in 1985. While it's possible that this malfunction is what led to the sickness that occurred on the island, personally, I think it's the other way around. The numbers glitch most likely affected the Cerberus, causing it to go berserk and eject people who weren't ready to be ejected. Even though 1985 is a bit before Danielle supposedly arrived on the island, assuming she's got her numbers wrong, (no pun intended) this could be what had killed her crew. After all, in her distress signal she says "it killed them … it killed them all." If this is the case, however, it opens another mystery as to why Danielle would later claim responsibility for their deaths (to Sayid). Unless she was the cause for the glitch to begin with, and her guilt has warped her memories. As with our own minds, in the simulated world, anything's possible.

Up to this point, you may be reading these theories and nodding your head for the most part but still are not fully convinced of the simulation solution. Well, allow me to drive the final nail into the coffin of skepticism to enable you to put any doubt to rest. If you're an avid *Lost* viewer, no doubt you've noticed that creepy clicking noise that the monster makes. It sorta sounds like a chikita-chik chickita-chik chickita-chik. It's a very mechanical sound—not very natural at all. Wanna know what that sound is from? Perhaps you've even found it to be familiar? Especially if you live in New York. What is it? According to producers, it's the sound of a receipt being printed out of a New York City taxicab. Pretty cool, you say, but how does that prove the simulation theory?

In and of itself, it proves nothing. Many sound effects featured in movies and TV shows are taken from real objects found in our environment. If you've ever watched that early *Star Wars* FX special, you saw how the sound designers came up with much of the sound effects of the movie from ordinary things like banging on telephone pole cables and the like. So what's the difference here? The sound had to come from somewhere, right? The difference is that when Rose first heard the sound of the monster during the pilot episode, she said that it sounded familiar to her … and Rose is from the Bronx. If Rose could recognize the taxi receipt noise, then that sound actually exists and doesn't originate naturally with the monster, making it an artificial thing to have its sound taken from something else. If the island were a real location, and therefore the monster a real, albeit possibly mechanical creature, why would someone need to give an artificial noise to it? You don't need to make a noise for a tank, or a car, or a lawn mower. These things have sounds of their own. But, if you create something within a program, you *do* have to create sounds for it, or else it would all be silent. Killing someone is the monster's last course of action. Before doing that, it hopes to intimidate, and it can't do that if it's silently sneaking up on people. Hence, the creepy taxi receipt noise. Anyone that's ever been in a NYC taxicab is already conditioned to be afraid of that noise. Paying by the second when you're stuck in New York traffic is a scary thing, indeed.

The Numbers

While I think I've already done a rather thorough job explaining the significance of the numbers, since that explanation is spread throughout several sections, I thought I'd just lay it all down here and further clarify some details. Basically, I believe that the numbers—4, 8, 15, 16, 23, and 42—are a bug or glitch in the system that resulted in them appearing far more often than mere chance would suggest, both on the island and in the castaways' flashbacks. As previously discussed, it is very likely that what happens on the island, as well as the events in many of the flashbacks, are simulations. They would need to be simulations to explain how the characters got to the island. This is why the numbers show up in the character's memories—because their memories are coming from the computer, which is infected with this glitch.

As mentioned in the previous section, the "malfunction" on the island happened in 1985. Therefore, any flashbacks we see before that time should not feature the numbers any more frequently than they normally would appear. To date, the only flashback we've seen that is supposed to have occurred before 1985 is the beginning of Ben's. During a scene from this flashback, young Ben disables the security fence code using the number 54439. Unlike the other random numbers that we see appearing on the island, this one is not made up of solely the infamous numbers sequence. The reason is most likely because the glitch hasn't happened yet, so the numbers were still relatively random.

The two "fours" may be an indicator of things to come, but they might also be purely random since none of the other numbers appear.

To counteract the glitch, DHARMA programmers created a system update of sorts that had to be applied from within the simulation. To keep the numbers from appearing so frequently, they were purposely plugged in within a controlled environment to balance out the system's need to create them randomly. This treatment involved several measures, including broadcasting the numbers from the radio tower (which had been done before Rousseau changed it), inserting them into a computer at the Swan station (the source of the glitch), and injecting a liquefied version of the numbers into the cyber-version of people within the system as an antidote to the sickness the numbers caused. The numbers were also permanently embedded in certain key locations throughout the island where they had been showing up the most frequently—such as on top of the Swan hatch. Apart from these instances, most of the occurrences of the numbers on the island were made by people within the simulation noticing that they existed. This explains the numbers in Rousseau's notes and on the blast door map in the Swan hatch. So it would seem that the system upgrade had succeeded in keeping the numbers at bay on the island, but accomplishing this within people's memories was a different story.

In flashbacks, the numbers show up constantly. Most notably, they all form the sequence of numbers Hurley plays to win the lottery. Individually, the numbers show up much more frequently. In fact, whenever a random number is supposed to be used, whether as a room number, price tag, speed gage, birth date, temperature, or number on a sports jersey, it usually involves one, or a combination of, the numbers. But remember, what we are seeing is not real memories—even if they are based on real events, they are the simulation's interpretation of the castaway's memories. Therefore, one of the numbers can be plugged in by the computer whenever a random number is needed. It's the same as when a Lostie gets someone plugged into their memory from another Lostie's experience if their memory of that person is unclear or if the memory is completely fabricated.

While all this is well and good, none of this explains why these specific numbers are used to represent the now infamous numbers sequence. At the 2005 Comic-Con, *Lost* executive producer Damon

Lindelof reportedly admitted that "we may never know what the numbers mean." Obviously, this statement pissed off a lot of fans, and so no one on the show has spoken a peep about the numbers since. I think what Damon was referring to, though, is the *specific* numbers used in the show, as opposed to their overall significance that I just theorized. Even if it's unlikely to ever be explained on the show, I believe there is a reason the writers chose the specific numbers they did. Let's explore some possibilities, shall we?

For starters, when developing the numbers, I feel like the creators wanted their total to be 108 no matter what they were. The reason is because the number 108 shows up many times within world religions, especially within Eastern religions. In Buddhism and Hinduism in particular, 108 has great significance. There are 108 beads on a mala, which is a string of beads Buddhists and Hindus use for counting chants when meditating. Buddhists also believe there are 108 defilements of the mind (or 108 ways one can get lost). Similarly, the bells at temples throughout Japan ring 108 times on New Year's Eve to rid the body of its 108 earthly desires and free it from evil. So 108 would seem to be a bad thing, perfect for the total of the numbers that might cause a glitch. Even if it's not necessarily bad, 108 might be powerful. In Judaism, eighteen is the numerical equivalent of life, and Jews often multiply it into various sums for gifts and the like. Multiply it six times, and you get 108. There are many more occurrences, but you get the point. 108 was the goal sum. But what of the rest of the numbers to be used to get there?

Well, four is a very natural number, so it was probably an obvious choice. There are four seasons, four elements (earth, air, fire, and water), and four central tenets of Buddhism known as the Four Noble Truths. I believe that eight and sixteen were then selected since, besides having their own spiritual and mythological meanings (Buddhist's Eightfold Path, Sweet Sixteen), each is the double of the next number (I'll get to fifteen in a moment). Next, twenty-three was chosen most likely because of its connection to the Illuminati and conspiracy theories. I'm not going to get into details here since there have been books and movies on this very subject (like the recent one with Jim Carrey called *The Number 23*). If you're interested, you'll find a wealth of information just by Googling "Illuminati 23." Suffice to say, twenty-three is a cult number that shows up frequently in many TV shows and movies. The same can be said of forty-two—which is "the answer to life, the universe, and everything" according to Douglas Adams in his book *The Hitchhiker's Guide to the Galaxy.* Due to the cult/nerd popularity of the book (one of my favorites), the number has been used countless times in a tribute to Adams and the story. For example, there was the English pop group Level 42, Fox Mulder's apartment number was forty-two, and if you type *the answer to life, the universe, and everything* into Google, you'll get "42" from the Google calculator.

Once the writers had five numbers, they probably decided to get one more so they'd have six. Why? I dunno. Possibly 'cause 666 is the number of the Beast, but more likely just because they wanted more than five digits. Since they knew they wanted the total to equal 108, they subtracted the total of the numbers they already had from that number and got fifteen. So fifteen became one of the numbers. Sure, I'm just guessing, but none of this really matters anyway. Regardless of what numbers the writer's chose, people would be wondering what their significance was. They could've just as easily picked 3, 7, 12, 13, 21, and 52 and gotten a total of 108 and lots of explanations as to what those numbers mean. In fact, there's probably an alternate dimension that exists right now where those *are* the numbers they chose, but that's a hypothesis for a different book.

While I'm taking the stance that the number sequence is a glitch and that the specific numbers themselves have no real relevance within the story, there is a scenario where I can see them playing an important role. This scenario involves my alternate theory where the Lost Island is, in fact, a computer running the earth that plans on wiping out its human virus inhabitants that are making it sick. Needing, perhaps, to have some humans around to complete its ecosystem, the computer decides to save certain individuals and so decides to bring some candidates to its shores. To make sure that these humans are worthy to be saved, it challenges them with certain tasks. Those who pass will seemingly be killed, but will actually be transported to a safe zone where they will survive the coming cataclysm. Of the humans that are left behind, they will be given a bonus series of clues that will tell them when the disaster is set to occur so that they might seek shelter. The date of that disaster will be April 8, 2015 at 4:23:42 PM, or 4/8/15 at

16:23:42 when expressed numerically in military time. Interestingly, the numbers do fit into a date and time arrangement. They could also fit into a location arrangement of longitude and latitude or a combination of time and location. While intriguing, I'm still sticking to my simulation theory, but again, this alternate theory *would* satisfy the mythology of the show.

More important than why the specific numbers are chosen to represent the numbers sequence is what the myth of the numbers is supposed to represent in our world. If the numbers are a glitch, what would be the equivalent in our so-called real lives? For the answer, we once again turn to *The Matrix*. (Okay, now this is getting creepy. For the second time since I began writing this book, Microsoft Word just "unexpectedly quit." The last time it crashed was also when I was writing about the numbers glitch. The universe has a funny way of giving us confirmations that we're on the right track.) Remember in *The Matrix* when Neo sees a black cat and then sees a similar one walk by, just like the first one? He attributes it to déjà vu, but Trinity explains that déjà vu is a glitch in the Matrix that happens when the programmers change something. It's pretty much the same thing here. The numbers are the glitch in the Lost Simulation, and they mythically represent our experience of déjà vu. But wouldn't that mean that we actually live in some sort of simulated world too? Could be …

Joop The Orangutan

What's up with Joop? According to *The Lost Experience* on-line adventure, Joop benefits from the Hanso Foundation's experiments by reaching the ripe old age of 105, making him the world's oldest orangutan. And besides Joop, what about all that other stuff in *The Lost Experience* and the Hanso Foundation TV ads (go to YouTube. com and type in "Hanso" to see some of their ads that ran during the regular season) that allude to similar life-extension experiments and other seemingly sci-fi discoveries? Seems like a whole helluva lotta stuff for the writers to keep track of. How will it all get resolved? Answer—it most likely won't. It's all BS, meant to throw you all off the scent, you nosey clue dogs, you! I believe they're all red herrings. The writers throw all that stuff out there as a distraction, leading viewers down a path meant to make us believe that *Lost* is about some kind of salvation for humanity (see my first, now rejected, theory). As stated earlier, I do believe that DHARMA's original plan was to conduct scientific research within the simulation (which may have included life-extending treatments and the like), but since the Hostiles took over, this work no longer seems to be a priority.

While the idea that *Lost* is actually about real-world experiments meant to save mankind is certainly intriguing and fits in with many of the clues the show has given us, my big problem with this is that it has nothing to do with why all the characters have issues. Sure, the writers could make up some convoluted theory, but it'll feel exactly like that—convoluted. Yes, it is *possible* that the island is real and that it's trying to collect a strong selection of humans to prevent mankind from going extinct. Great idea—but why chose so many selfish people? Unless the island is evil and plans on killing off the good guys it doesn't select. No, that would contradict the myth. Well, how about if the island is taking problem candidates, hoping it can correct their lives and get mankind back on track with its destiny? As discussed, USA's *The 4400* has already gone this route. Maybe the *Lost* gang is part of another experiment to see if mankind is even worth saving in the first place, and the Others are, in fact, aliens. Sorry, not buying it. I would think that experiments to see if man is worth saving would have been done *before* the experiments to actually save them. If this ends up being the writer's solution, I'm going to start a petition to have their ending annulled and mine produced and aired as the real ending.

Other Loose Ends

So now that I've cleared up those twenty mysteries, there are only about fifty or sixty more to go. What's up with the black and white rocks that were found in one of the skeleton's pockets? How about the "Hurley Bird"—the bird that squawked Hurley's name? What did those hieroglyphics mean when the numbers in the Swan station went down to zero? What about the supply drop? The pillar of smoke that the Others set off on the island? The Christian symbols? The psalms on Mr. Eko's staff? The connections with old songs? Claire's baby? Sun's lover? What's up with everything else? Well … I'll leave those answers up to you.

Oh, I've got my theories, and I think that by using what I've already discussed in this book, you could figure out most of them on your own and probably come up with some ideas that are even better. Just remember that a lot of the hints people are looking at are simply the writers having fun—giving us tasty but meaningless morsels to uncover that only serve to throw us off the trail so smart-asses like myself won't go figuring it all out and blabbing it to the world. The perfect example of this is the *Lost*-inspired novel called *Bad Twin*—a supposedly non-fiction book written by a fictional author, which pretty much makes it all completely fiction. The story follows a private investigator who's hired to track down one of the missing twins from the very wealthy Widmore family (owners of Widmore Corporation, which funds Hanso, which funds DHARMA). The book's author is the fictitious Gary Troup (possibly Stephen King), who supposedly died aboard Oceanic Flight 815 and whose name, interestingly enough, is an anagram for "purgatory." Since the release of the book, *Lost* has pretty much killed the purgatory theory (particularly with its third season finale), so the anagram is just another example of the writers trying to throw us off the trail.

From a more mythological perspective, all these mini-mysteries that *Lost* continually bombards viewers with are simply meant to keep them distracted from the real questions—just as the material world keeps us distracted from the real questions here. Sometimes, the writers don't even need to try to create these distractions. We just do it ourselves, overanalyzing details of the show that aren't meant to be analyzed at all. I mean, you can't believe how much work people have put into trying to figure out some of the show's mysteries. Trust me, if the answers are that complicated, the average viewer isn't going to be able to understand them.

That being said, there are some connections and hints in the show that the writers actually have put in as clues, but these usually reveal insights to characters and themes rather than anything about the overall mystery. An example of just such a clue deals with Ethan Rom. He's the guy that the Losties thought was a fellow crash survivor, but turned out to be an Other who abducted Claire. His name provided the tip-off—Ethan Rom is an anagram for an "Other man." Even more intriguing than the clues the writers put in on purpose, are those that

152

they themselves probably didn't even know were in there. The fact that Hanso is an anagram for Noah's may be just such an example, as are the many objects that happen to form crosses in nearly every episode. These are quite possibly nothing but happy accidents that wind up in the show purely by coincidence. Then again, since there are no coincidences, these little nuggets just may be the mythology of the show weaving its way into the story's inner matrix so that it might somehow connect to our subliminal minds.

Like I said, I think *Lost* is working on a deeper level than its creators realize. They've created something that's taken on a life of its own, while simultaneously swallowing up the lives of many of its viewers. That's not to say that the show is a waste of time by any means. Au contraire, thanks to its subliminal and subconscious messages, you are now probably wiser about life's mysteries than you were before you began watching the show. Perhaps a part of your brain has been activated that previously had lain dormant. And perhaps this part will be a catalyst for a chain of events leading to your mental and possibly biological evolution that will enable you and your loved ones to survive the coming apocalypse and breed the next species of humankind. Or, perhaps that's just J. J. Abrams next show. Or, perhaps it'll be yours.

Where *Lost* Should Go from Here

Well, that pretty much explains everything. One of the reasons I'm so confident in the simulation theory is because all of *Lost*'s mysteries can be explained by it so perfectly. That's not to say that another theory couldn't do so as well, but I think it would still have to use the same "life as illusion" myth that the simulation theory is based upon. Using a bad idea I mentioned earlier as an example, maybe it'll turn out that the Others are really aliens ... and they have been testing the Losties to see if mankind is worthy of being saved ... and that the island is their ship where they are conducting their experiments. Even if all of this is the case, everything would *still* have to be an illusion since nothing would be as it appeared. It's all the same myth. In one way or another, the Losties are living in a reality outside of their own. That's the mythology of the show, the rest is just details. Once you have that basic mythic element, everything else can plug right in. I think the simulation theory works the best. The show creators may have a different resolution—but even so, the symbolism, analogies, archetypes, and general mythology will still remain the same as what I interpret here. In other words, even if the simulation theory is completely wrong, Jack and Locke are still the heroes, the whispers still represent our gut instinct, and we should still seek out the clues the universe gives us to help us fulfill our destinies. None of that will change, no matter what the solution ends up being.

Just for the record, even though I believe I have a viable solution, I'll still be watching—just with a different eye. An eye looking to see what correlates with the simulation theory and what seems to not quite fit. I'm especially interested to see how the writers will go about explaining the many unresolved mysteries and what their version of the answers will be. Will the solutions be revealed by using character flashbacks and flash-forwards? Will they bring us directly outside the computer simulation (time-warping island, alien spaceship, whatever) and show us what's really going on? Will they use one long flashback as I've described and take us back to the beginning of the DHARMA project, possibly using one of the DHARMA doctors to explain everything to a recuperating Jack? Or will they come up with some method that's completely different altogether?

Judging from the third season finale, it looks as though the mysteries will all be answered piece by piece with flashbacks and flash-forwards, fitting them together like a jigsaw puzzle. Problem is, this may get awfully confusing after a while as the audience tries to figure out not only what is going on but when it's happening in the storyline. There are a lot of questions that still remain unanswered, and somehow they have to all be resolved around the time that the main mystery is revealed, so as not to give too much away. How the creators plan on doing this is very interesting to me. And yet, something tells me that they are very interested in resolving this conundrum themselves.

In a way, I think the writers for *Lost* have kind of written themselves into a corner by building up the mystery of the show as the end-all be-all. Personally, I think that once you know what's going on is when the show can really start getting good. It's at that point when we see how the mysterious elements of the show all fit together. How and why everyone comes together the way they do. That's why I thought that a season cliffhanger should have Jack getting "killed" and then waking up only to see his dad. He'd finally be outside of the computer simulation, but we wouldn't know that yet.

Then, when the next season started, the story could go back to the beginning of the DHARMA Initiative, explaining how the whole project evolved. After only a few episodes, we'd slowly begin to realize that the *Lost* world is only a simulation, but we still wouldn't know how everything fits into it, and *that's* what would keep us watching. How do the polar bears get there? Why does the young Danielle Rousseau come into the program, and what happens to the rest of her team? How does Leonard Simms come to know the numbers? When and how does Kelvin show up? What about the original Henry Gale? And the Others? What *really* happens between Desmond and Libby? How is it that Libby is in a mental hospital? If the Losties aren't really in Australia, how do they come to hear about the program, why do they sign up, and what is the reality of their lives? I think it would be very interesting to see their *real* stories. Does Walt actually have powers? Does Sawyer really shoot the guy he thinks is the real Sawyer? Is Jack's dad really dead? Even knowing the truth about the main mystery of *Lost,* you'd still tune in to get answers to these and other questions. I know I would.

After this series of flashback episodes solves most of the mysteries, we could then return to my proposed scenario of Jack waking up and seeing his father. Only now, in addition to his dad, he also sees Boone, Shannon, Mr. Eko, Libby, Ana Lucia, Charlie, (once again, *The Wizard of Oz* myth) and whoever else had supposedly died or left the island— maybe even Michael and Walt. Imagine the drama there between Michael, Libby, and Ana Lucia. You could have a whole spin-off series on that alone! But getting back to Jack, his dad, along with the rest of the gang, could explain to him what has happened, and as he regains consciousness, he would start to remember everything himself. But then what? Would he demand to go back into the system to tell everyone else the truth? Would he go back in for further treatment, perhaps with a new batch of patients? Or, as we saw in his flash-forward, would he attempt to get his life back together only to discover that he is not only not cured, he is worse?

Once I saw how messed up Jack was in the flash-forward episode, my feeling was that he would not "die" on the island but would somehow escape before conquering his demons. As I've said, I believe that those who legitimately die in the simulation after resolving their issues, like Mr. Eko, Boone, and Charlie, are cured in the outside world, while those who don't, like Michael (and possibly Jack and Kate), are not. Cured or not, how the various characters turn out is definitely something most fans would want to see, and this explains why the *Lost* writers opted for the flash-forwards. They are probably the best way to show what happens to all the characters after they get off the island, without revealing exactly what the island is.

Apparently, the *Lost* creators felt that once the big mystery is revealed, audiences will lose interest. For this reason, the main mystery probably won't be solved until the end. I'm assuming that season four will continue to utilize the flash-forwards, possibly focusing on what became of Michael and Walt, as well as continuing Jack and Kate's story—if not all the Losties. While intriguing, this method could get confusing. That's why I prefer letting the audience in on the big mystery first, and then using one long flashback to fill in the remaining blanks. This would enable viewers to finally know what the island really is, and to watch as the remaining characters try to figure it out. So the characters would still be lost, but we would no longer be.

The way I'd love to see the show finally conclude would involve seeing all the main characters back to their real lives. Some have been successfully treated, some have improved somewhat, and some are back to their old tricks. Just as we think the final episode is about to end, however, the camera pulls back to reveal *yet another* veil of reality. It would turn out that even the characters' real lives aren't real after all, but an illusionary realm as seen from the perspective of the spiritual world. From this viewpoint, we see the characters' souls controlling their respective "real-world" bodies much like video game characters. As the screen turns to black and the words *Lost* appear in bold white type on the screen, a tiny part of us is left wondering whether or not our world is, in fact, actually real. Whether, much like *Lost*, the world we live in is also an illusion, and we are here to rise above our own inner challenges, defeat the shapeless monsters around us, put together the clues to solve our own mysteries, meet the people who are meant to be in our lives, learn from them, and fulfill our destinies. Perhaps we really are all lost in an illusionary world, and *Lost* has gotten us one step closer to being found.

Now What?
How the Wisdom of *Lost* Can Apply to Your Life

So, now you know the answers to all the big questions—at least about *Lost*. Then again, as I just pointed out, you might also have some of the answers to life too. All you need to do is look deeper into the myth. Since *Lost* is a microcosm of our world, all the rules that apply to it should also apply on some level to our reality. For example, in the episode "The Man from Tallahassee," Ben describes to Locke a magic box that is located somewhere on the island. He goes on to say that whatever you imagine or wish to be in the box would appear once you open it. Being lost in the illusionary world, Locke takes the reference literally. However, the magic box is not an actual box that physically exists, but a metaphor for the island's ability to make the wants or needs of its inhabitants materialize. Ben even admits this in a later episode.

In our world, this metaphor relates to the immensely popular spiritual principle known as the Law of Attraction, which has helped make books like *The Secret* such an amazing success. Put simply, the Law of Attraction states that our mind attracts the events we experience in life. So if you think positive thoughts, your mind will attract positive events into your life, and if you think negative thoughts, negative events will likely occur. Using this wisdom, we can make our wishes more likely to become realities by training our mind to focus on our dreams. The mythology of *Lost* demonstrates this principle by showing us how the power of the island enables people to get what they need from within the simulation program—especially if it will help them fulfill their destinies. In Locke's case, the island brings his father to him so that he can "kill" the one thing that is holding him back from releasing his true potential.

While all this universal wish-granting stuff may seem like science-fiction, there actually is a lot of theoretical science out there that could explain how thoughts creating realities could work beyond simple magical thinking. According to some interpretations of quantum theory, there are an infinite number of possibilities occurring right at this moment, and our thoughts bring us to the ones we believe ourselves to be in. By this definition, we are not causing our wishes to appear; we are simply leaping into a reality where they already exist. Yes, this may seem complicated, and that's why *Lost* attempts to explain it in terms we can understand—a computer simulation. When we clear a level in any video game, from the character's perspective, it brings about a whole other reality that didn't previously exist. Yet we, the players, know that this new level has already been programmed into the game. In fact, every action the computer game character could possibly take has already been programmed. As eerie as it sounds, our lives may work similarly.

What if we really are all living in a computer program—or at least, something that acts like one—and the point of our lives is to correct certain flaws or issues we have in order to move to the next level? This theme is not only what *Lost* is all about, but is also the basis of most of the world's religions. In many Eastern philosophies, we are reincarnated in order to work out unresolved issues from previous lives. According to Christianity, those who follow the teachings of Jesus will go to heaven when they die, while those who don't will go to hell. Many Jews believe that, by following the commandments of the Torah, they will be chosen to share the world with the Messiah when he finally arrives. Recognize a pattern? While constantly bickering about what sets them apart, most of the world's religions seem to agree that there is something beyond the material world we live in and that we are here to challenge ourselves in order to one day get there. So if there's another reality beyond our own, and it's a reality that we're all meant to strive for, then ... where exactly are we now?

This world—this island Earth that we've all grown so accustomed to—is but an illusion created to help us challenge ourselves and have experiences as separate beings. This is not possible in the other realm, where we know we are all one. So this illusionary world has been created to make it possible. We are still all one—we just don't know it because of the illusion of separateness. I'm not making this stuff up. A lot of it comes from ancient mystical beliefs. If you can accept it and go with the flow of what life throws at you—striving to be proactive and reach your destiny—then you'll do well. If not, life will be a constant struggle. What might make it easier is the belief that there is nowhere we have to go to. We are all meant to be here. It is not necessary to live our lives in order to be rewarded in some heavenly existence—we should live our lives in order to bring heaven to *this* existence, now. Yes, life may be but a video game, but isn't the point of video games to challenge ourselves, experience new adventures, and have fun? Isn't this what our newest myths are attempting to communicate?

If you can accept that the world we live in is an illusion, you can be like Locke and look out for the clues that will help you to fulfill your destiny and then challenge yourself to get there, or you can be like Jack and resist changing, react negatively to the challenges life throws at you, wind up miserable, and then have to come back and try again in your next life. The other option is to be like the traitor in *The Matrix* who decides to live it up in the illusionary world and surround himself with nothing but material pleasures. Of course, this guy is eventually shot, because people who focus only on the illusion of materialism will eventually have nothing because that's what the illusion is—nothing. It's amazing how much you can learn from TV and movies when you start to decipher their mythological messages.

Spawned most recently by the success of *The Matrix*, there have been a lot of movies, books, and TV shows of late that have explored the "life as illusion" mythology that I've based my entire *Lost* theory on. For whatever reason, the time has come for this spiritual truth to reintroduce itself to our collective consciousness. So the world's creative shamans—having tapped into this energy—are interpreting it for the masses. In other words, the world's storytellers and artists have been receiving the same mental download so we can all learn the truth about our existence and get an upgrade to Humanity 2.0. (The myths for *The X-Men, Heroes, The 4400,* and countless others are aligned with this "humanity upgrade" theory—all of them focusing on the next evolutionary advancements for mankind. Unfortunately, most of them also involve major catastrophes, as though we'll need one to grow to the next level.) Why are we getting these messages now? Perhaps because we are at last ready to believe them and act accordingly.

Knowing that we are all one, there would be no need for war, since we'd all ultimately want the same thing. There would be no poverty or hunger, since we'd all be more open to sharing with other members of our spiritual body. Knowing that everything happens for a reason and that the universe drops us clues, we'd be more inclined to search for these clues in our own life and interpret them so that we might successfully fulfill our destinies. I feel like I'm doing that right now by writing this book. And you are being given some clues about what your destiny might be by reading it. In effect, this will set in motion a chain reaction, which will lead to your receiving more clues and meeting more people meant to guide you on your path. And perhaps you already even know what that path is.

In life, it often does seem as though we have a certain path that we are meant to follow. When Desmond tries to change his, he isn't really able to. This is a lesson for our real lives. Not that we are helpless and have no control, but that there are certain things that are just meant to happen—and will happen—and the way in which they do is our choice. We can live life the easy way, or the hard way. When we step off our path, the universe gives us hints or connections to help us get back on. If we've really wandered away, then we are forcefully shoved by major life changes meant to take us in a much different direction. Whenever these major life changes happen, it's a sign that we are going the wrong way, and the universe is helping us to make the correction. While at the time of these traumatic events we may feel completely fearful, depressed, or angry, more times than not we will be better off in the long run. As they say, "Out of rejection comes direction," or "Pain pushes you until the vision pulls you," or, the most famous of these sayings, "When God closes one door, He opens another." So don't stare at the door that's just shut in your face—move on. There's something much better waiting for you; all you have to do is start walking toward it. So yes, you must act.

While there is a lot of truth to the Law of Attraction, many people have oversimplified the principles by which it works. The world isn't going to hand us our wishes on a silver platter simply by our wishing it so. We must act—overcoming our own bad habits and fears—in order to reach our dreams. This is another valuable lesson that has been illustrated on *Lost*. In the episode "Tricia Tanaka Is Dead," Hurley finds an old DHARMA van and, despite having faith, is unable to get it started. However, Hurley does not give up. He so believes that he can get the old van to start that he decides to risk his life in the process. So, for the second attempt, he and Charlie get into the van and ride it down a steep hill toward some jagged rocks. Just before the van is about to collide into the stones, he turns the ignition again, and this time it starts, enabling Hurley to turn the wheel and avoid certain disaster. But why does it work this time and not the first time? Because Hurley has taken a leap of faith. He isn't just *thinking* that an action will work, he is acting with the full expectation that it will—and this expectation is in line with his destiny. Later, Hurley uses the van to save Bernard, Sayid, and Jin from being executed by the Others. This is important to note. The belief has to be in line with your destiny. If I believe I can fly and jump off a building, unless my destiny is to be Superman, I'm going to fall. Your belief must be in line with your destiny, which will always be for the greater good.

This is the true meaning of the leap of faith myth, which is repeated throughout history. According to mystical interpretations of the Bible, Moses does not wave his arms to split the Reed (Red) Sea. He walks into it until it is above his head, fully expecting it to split. Just as he is about to drown, the waves part, setting the precedent for the leap of faith—an action taken for the greater good, based on the belief that something *must* work.

While risking one's life is the most powerful example of the leap of faith, thankfully it is not necessary in order to be effective. We just need to put ourselves out there by taking the kind of risks that will enable us to reach our dreams. The true power of the Law of Attraction is that you need to live as though your desires have already occurred. You need to make room for them to enter your life. To wait around for your ship to come in is not truly believing. You must quit your crappy job, dump your partner who doesn't believe in you, move to a better location, invest in your new business—whatever it is, you must act, not simply wish. When you wish for something, you are in effect acting as though you do not already have it, and this is what is duplicated by the Law of Attraction: your need to wish for something because you don't already have it. So don't just wish for your dreams to be fulfilled, know that they will be, and act accordingly. Yet another excellent life-truth subliminally demonstrated to us on *Lost,* the Bible, and a million other myths.

All of these mythological messages may seem far-fetched, but what if they are true? What if life really is nothing more than an illusion, making us but vehicles for God to experience all of life's adventures? Or, what if we are all truly human, but from another dimension where we pay to be in this very realistic computer simulation so we can overcome our issues from that other realm? Considering we're still here, I guess we're not doing too well. Then again, with over six billion of us on this planet, we're all in good company. And it isn't even necessary for *everyone* to come to accept the reality—or unreality—of our situation in order for us all to overcome it. Once 51 percent of us have seen the light, it'll tip the entire scale. It's called a critical mass. And right now, it's critical that we get a mass of people on board with these beliefs so we can start moving in the right direction. The writers of *Lost* have done their part. I've begun doing my share. Now, it's your turn.

The biggest irony about *Lost* is that it's about a group of people in a simulated world who don't know that they are in a simulated world being watched by an audience who will eventually learn that the characters are in a simulated world but will probably still not realize they, themselves, are also living in a simulated world. Your eyes are now opened to the universal truth of *Lost* that resonated with your soul, causing you to feel inexplicably drawn to its mystery. A mystery that a piece of you longed to be a part of, and strangely enough, turned out to be something you were a part of all along (you could've gone home at any time, Dorothy; you just had to click your heels and envision it). All of us have been lost. Lost in an illusionary world of materialism where our lives have come to be valued by what we have, rather than what we are. We are all connected. We are all here to improve ourselves and to help others do the same for themselves. Everything happens for a reason, and the clues are all around us. Yes, as you had suspected, *Lost* is much more than a show. It's the way life really works. Now we must go beyond just watching it and start living it.

Before we begin, however, we can all learn a lesson from the mistakes of Mr. Locke—don't get so caught up in the clues that you start to rely on them for all your answers. They are meant to guide, not control. So just as you shouldn't get obsessed with the clues of the show, don't get obsessed with the clues in your own life. Look for the signs. Listen for the whispers. But then make up your own mind about what they all mean, because ultimately you control your own fate. Yes, we all have a destiny, but there are multiple paths we can take to get there. With some, you may run into a monster, a ghost from your past, or even a polar bear, but don't fret; these are but challenges that are put in your way so that you can rise above them. The more that you successfully conquer, the stronger you'll become, and the more likely you'll be to get where you want to go.

You got a whole lot more than you bargained for when you picked up this book, ay? You were looking for commentary on a mysterious TV show and wound up with an explanation to the mysteries of the universe. I hope you found what you were looking for and will discover and accomplish your destiny, whatever it may be. May the lessons you've been absorbing from *Lost* now reside in your consciousness where you can act on them. And may they result in our world coming to realize that the mythology of *Lost* is not mythology at all. But the truth of our existence.

See ya in another life.

Sources

Celestial Weather. http://celestialweather.com/ftp/100206.html.

Lost: The Complete First Season. September, 2005.

The Lost Experience. http://www.thelostexperience.com/.

Lostpedia.com. http://lostpedia.com/wiki/Whisper_transcripts.

Peacock, Thomas Love. *Headlong Hall.* London, England: Aldine House, 1891.

Plato. Trans. Jowett, B. *Plato's The Republic.* New York: The Modern Library, 1941.

Notes

1. Dictionary.com. http://dictionary.reference.com/browse/myth.

2. Weinstein, Simcha. *Up, Up, and Oy Vey!: How Jewish History, Culture, and Values Shaped the Comic Book Superhero.* Baltimore, Maryland: Leviathan Press, 2006.

3. Fleischer, Jeff. "Superman's Other Secret Identity." World Jewish Digest. Online. July 25, 2006.

4. HollywoodJesus.com. http://www.hollywoodjesus.com/superman. htm.

5. Dictionary.com. http://dictionary.reference.com/ search?r=2&q=archetype

6. Agnes, Michael. *Webster's New World College Dictionary, Fourth Edition.* Cleveland, Ohio: Wiley Publishing, Inc., 2004.

7. Dos Santos, Kristin. "*Lost* Redux: Damon Lindelof Breaks 'Radio Silence' to Reveal Why Charlie Died and More." E! Online. May 23, 2007.

8. Philosophy Professor. http://www.philosophyprofessor.com/ philosophers/david-hume.php

9. —. http://www.philosophyprofessor.com/philosophers/jean-jacques-rousseau.php.

10. Lostpedia. http://lostpedia.com/wiki/Black_rock.

11. Baby Names World. http://www.babynamesworld.com/
meaning_of_Nadia.html.

12. SciFi2U. http://www.scifi2u.com/index.php?option=com_
content&task=blogcategory&id= 130&Itemid=365.

13. Jensen, Jeff. "The Isle Files." EW.com. January 31, 2007.

14. "*Lost* Producers: We Won't End Like *Sopranos*." CNN.com.
June 14, 2007.

15. Jensen, Jeff. "Flash-Forward Thinking." EW.com. May 29, 2007.

16. Lang, Silke Berit. "The Impact of Video Systems on
Architecture." Dissertation, Swiss Federal Institute of Technology
Zurich, 2004. p. 53.

17. Bentham, Jeremy. Ed. Miran Bozovic. *The Panopticon Writings*.
London, England: Verso, 1995. p. 29–95.

18. Jensen. "Flash-Forward Thinking."

Printed in the United States
130647LV00004B/2/P